CONSENT, RIGHTS AND CHOICES IN HEALTH CARE FOR CHILDREN AND YOUNG PEOPLE

CONSENT, RIGHTS AND CHOICES IN HEALTH CARE FOR CHILDREN AND YOUNG PEOPLE

British Medical Association
BMA House
Tavistock Square
London
WC1H 9JP

© BMJ Books 2001
BMJ Books is an imprint of the BMJ Publishing Group

First published in 2001
by BMJ Books, BMA House, Tavistock Square,
London WC1H 9JR

Second impression 2001
Third impression 2003

www.bmjbooks.com

British Library Cataloguing in Publication Data

A catalogue record for this book is available from the British Library

ISBN 0-7279-1228-3

Typeset by FiSH Books, London
Printed and bound by JW Arrowsmith, Bristol

Contents

v

CONTENTS

CONTENTS

CONTENTS

List of cases

Cases before the European Court and Commission of Human Rights

List of statutes and regulations

LIST OF CASES AND STATUTES

Membership of the Steering Group

Mr Allan Levy QC   Barrister and Recorder (Chairman)

Dr Priscilla Alderson   Reader in Childhood Studies, Institute of Education, London

Mr Phil Bates   Lecturer in Law, King's College, London

Dr Ieuan Davies   Specialist Registrar (Paediatrics), Ysbyty Glan Clwyd, North Wales; Member of the BMA's Medical Ethics Committee

Dr Donna Dickenson   Leverhulme Reader in Medical Ethics and Law, Imperial College, London

Dr Elaine Gadd   Senior Medical Officer (Medical Ethics), Department of Health

Professor David Harvey   Consultant Paediatrician, London

Ms Rachel Hodgkin   Principal Policy Officer and Clerk to the All Party Parliamentary Group for Children, National Children's Bureau to 1998; Consultant on Children's Rights and Policy

Mr Peter Honig   Family Therapist and Social Worker, Cambridge

Ms Claire Johnston   Family and Medical Lawyer, Official Solicitor's Office

Professor Neil McIntosh   Paediatrician, Edinburgh; Chairman of the Royal College of Paediatrics and Child Health's Ethics Committee

MEMBERSHIP OF THE STEERING GROUP

Mr Jonathan Montgomery   Reader in Health Care Law, University of Southampton; Chairman of the Southampton Community Health Services NHS Trust

Mr Michael Nicholls   Barrister, Official Solicitor's Office 1996–1998; 1 Mitre Court Buildings

Professor John Pearce   Emeritus Professor of Child and Adolescent Psychiatry, University of Nottingham

Professor Sir Michael Rutter   Professor of Developmental Psychopathology, Institute of Psychiatry, King's College, London

Dr Michael Wilks   Forensic Medical Examiner, London; Chairman of the BMA's Medical Ethics Committee

Editorial Board

The BMA is grateful to the following for their help: Ms Susan Attwood, Mr William Bingley, Mr James Dickson, Dr Ruth Gilbert, Sister Mary Goodwin, Mr Tony Harbour, Ms Lucy Heath, Professor J Stuart Horner, Dr Vincent Leach, Dr Frank Wells, the Royal College of Nursing and the United Kingdom Central Council for Nursing, Midwifery and Health Visiting. We also thank all those who gave written and oral evidence, particularly Dr Mark Berelowitz, Professor Elizabeth Fradd, Professor Alan Glasper, Ms Rachel Haggarty, Professor Ian Kennedy, Dr Vic Larcher and Mr Justice Munby.

Introduction

The reason for the book

This book addresses the ethical issues to do with treating children and young people most commonly raised by doctors. The British Medical Association has always received many enquiries from doctors about ethical and legal aspects of examining and treating children and young people. The flow of such enquiries increased during the 1990s and continues to rise. A range of diverse factors contributed to this. Part of the growth in queries can doubtless be attributed to increased awareness of children's autonomy and the importance of health professionals providing young patients, as well as their parents, with clear information. Changing perceptions of the rights of children and young people also raises questions about the role of parents and others with parental responsibility, particularly in relation to decisions about treatment for competent adolescents. Health professionals have always had to cope with exceptional cases where major disagreements about treatment arise between competent young patients and their families but the growing emphasis on listening to the personal preferences of all patients has made some such cases appear harder to resolve. The boundaries of confidentiality, both in terms of the rights of individuals and in terms of the family's privacy, also generate a substantial number of questions.

The involvement of children and young people in procedures that are not intended primarily for the benefit of their own health, such as medical research or tissue donation from living child donors has been another area of enquiry. In addition, in the late 1990s and in 2000, high profile public inquiries such as that into the past activities of doctors at centres including the Bristol Royal Infirmary, the North Staffordshire Hospital Trust and

INTRODUCTION

Liverpool's Alder Hey Hospital drew attention to a need to re-examine and publish clear guidance on some aspects of practice and to clarify the standards expected of doctors. Such inquiries highlighted past failures on the part of some practitioners to provide transparency, accountability and adequate assessment in relation to the application of new or risky procedures for very sick babies. Among other things, these tragic cases raised awareness within the profession about the manner in which any proposed innovative procedure, the details thereof and its inherent risks, should be explained to parents. Such cases contributed to the already widespread awareness of the importance of effective and sensitive communication skills for all health professionals. They also emphasised the need for more effective audit and assessment of outcomes, as well as highlighting the ethical obligations of colleagues to take action in respect of inadequate standards and poorly performing doctors. Similarly it became clear that, in the past, health professionals had not talked openly or adequately to bereaved parents about issues such as the retention of their deceased child's tissue for research purposes. As a result of such inquiries, some new guidance has been issued or is in preparation and this is referenced in relevant chapters of this book. For information about guidance since this book was written, please see the BMA's website at the address given below.

The law

The queries consistently raised by doctors reveal some uncertainty about aspects of the law regarding consent and refusal of treatment in relation to children and young people. Therefore, this guidance sets out the current legal position. The legal provisions in England, Wales and Northern Ireland are discussed in chapter 2. The law in Scotland is discussed in chapter 3. The rest of the book covers all UK jurisdictions and considers recent case law as well as statute in this area and some illustrative examples of relevant legal cases are included in most chapters. These examples, however, should not be seen as *necessarily* indicating how the courts would decide future cases but they are helpful in demonstrating the kinds of circumstances in which review by a court may be needed. Different legal arguments may be made in future on issues of rights following the enactment of the Human Rights Act 1998, which some commentators predict will increasingly focus attention on individual rights.

INTRODUCTION

In October 2000, as a result of the Human Rights Act, rights contained in the European Convention on Human Rights became part of UK law. The long term impact of this legislation on the health service and medical practice is, as yet, open to debate but it is something that health professionals need to take into account.[1] Guidance from the Home Office's Human Rights Task Force indicates how Article 8, for example, which includes the right to respect for the individual's private and family life, covers a vast range of issues, including the right to consent to medical treatment, parental custody of children and the use of information about individuals.[2] More broadly within society, the Act may come to affect the manner in which people think about individual rights, including those of children and young people. At the second reading of the then Human Rights Bill in the House of Lords in 1997, the Lord Chancellor, Lord Irvine, said this piece of legislation would "bring human rights home ... Our courts will develop human rights throughout society. A culture of awareness of human rights will develop".[3]

A number of the rights set out in the Act could form the basis of challenges to the actions or inaction of public authorities such as NHS trusts. When acting in their capacity as NHS staff, the acts or omissions of doctors and other health service employees could also be challenged under the Act. Advice to the BMA suggests that in fact all doctors, including those in private practice, may be bound by the legislation. In any event, the BMA advises all doctors to follow the Human Rights Act as a matter of good practice.

The following rights may be of particular relevance to medical treatment, including mental health care: the right to life (Article 2); the right not to be subjected to inhuman or degrading treatment (Article 3); the right to liberty and security (Article 5); the right to a fair hearing (Article 6); the right to respect for private and family life (Article 8) and the right not to suffer discrimination in relation to any of the other basic rights (Article 14). Lawyers in all disciplines need to be familiar with the implications of the Act.[4] As yet, how the rights will be used in practice remains very much a matter of speculation. BMA guidance on the implications of the Human Rights Act for medical practice is available on its website.

At the time of finalising this book in 2000, no specific assistance regarding children's consent to medical treatment was available from cases that have been decided in the past in

Strasbourg by the European Court (or Commission) of Human Rights. Nevertheless, it is reasonable to suppose that the Convention rights may well be used to support further the right to self-determination of competent young people. In such cases, it is important that health authorities and health professionals seek specific legal advice if a novel rights dimension is relied upon.

The aim of the book

The aim of the book is to provide guidance that is as clear and as practical as possible, drawing on advice already published by other reputable bodies. Because it reflects their questions, it is intended primarily for health professionals but has also been drafted to be accessible to patients, their families and other people with an interest in these issues. The book discusses the current ethical approach to consent, refusal and confidentiality in respect of provision of health care to children and young people. It also summarises the law on these same issues, identifies areas where the legal position is unclear and offers advice in such circumstances.

In order to get a rounded debate on the practical problems and informed opinion about solutions, the BMA invited some leading experts in this field to form a steering group. The membership is given below. The group took written and oral evidence from a wide range of contributors about the management of both routine and exceptional cases. One aim of this book is to show how the same ethical principles that underpin good routine practice apply equally in many of the hard and unusual cases. Although practice must not be driven by exceptional, particularly complex cases, these inevitably challenge health professionals and families and need to be taken into account. Therefore, attention is given in the book both to the accepted principles of daily practice and to the relatively rare cases where profound disagreements arise and conflict has to be managed in a way that maximises benefit and minimises harm. We also draw attention to the way in which interpretations of commonly used concepts such as "benefit", "harm" and "best interests" have changed to reflect the importance placed on individual patients' views of what would be of benefit to them.

Terminology in the book

Terminology in this area of medical practice is particularly fraught for various reasons.

Best interests: Some frequently used terms are vague and open to broad interpretation. Decision making by reference to a patient's "best interests", for example, sounds reassuring but could be interpreted as authorising any procedure that is likely to improve physical health. At various places in the book (and particularly in chapter 1), we seek to demonstrate that patients' interests are not only defined in terms of physical benefit — vital as that usually is — but also in terms of what best accommodates their other needs.

Benefit and harm: Medicine is clearly founded on the notion of providing benefit. Inevitably, however, any analyses of concepts such as "benefit" and "harm" raise complex moral questions that, although fascinating in themselves, may not provide practical assistance to practitioners and patients. Nevertheless, the book seeks to show briefly how the understanding of concepts such as best interests, benefit and harm have widened very much beyond the relatively straightforward measurement of purely physical health indicators to include concepts such as psychological and social harm. In brief, in exceptional cases, overriding an informed minor's wishes may produce a health benefit but at the cost of other kinds of harm, including loss of trust and a breakdown in cooperation. Clearly, this does not mean that health professionals or parents can never act against a minor's wishes but rather that the full dimensions of the harms and benefits that flow from the decision need to be carefully weighed by all those involved in making it, including the child. While flagging up the complexities involved, however, our principal aim remains the provision of clear and practical guidance in order to identify a way forward in such cases.

Children and young people: As we discuss in chapter 1, the term "child" is frequently used to cover everyone from birth to the age of 18 (those under the age of majority or "minors") but does not reflect the diversity that is found within that particular population. Such terminology can be a source of irritation to young adults, some of whom lead very independent, working lives before the age of 18. We considered categorising young patients as babies, toddlers, pre-school children, children, adolescents and young people. A disadvantage of this approach, however, is that it appears to run contrary to a very basic point that we repeatedly emphasise in the book, which is the fact that all children and young people are individuals. They are constantly changing, developing and maturing and should not, where it is avoidable, be routinely pigeon-holed into particular groups. To do so is to reinforce often erroneous assumptions about particular individuals' levels of understanding and participation.

Understanding, personal experience and maturity are key issues in decision making but they are attributes that individuals acquire at differing rates (although, clearly, some generalisations can be usefully made, as we discuss in chapter 5). Because individuals within this population are constantly changing, it is important to emphasise that rigid blueprints and fixed assumptions about maturity and immaturity should be avoided. Throughout the book we stress that opinions about patients' abilities need to be constantly reassessed and related to a particular decision rather than to the labels or descriptions attached to patients. Generally, we have preferred the terms "children" for patients up to age 11 and "young people" for those aged 12 and over, although "minors" is occasionally used as a useful shorthand way of covering both. It is usually self-evident in the context of each chapter whether babies, very young children or more mature individuals are the subject of discussion. Clearly, most health professionals are well accustomed to dealing with issues of mental competence and, on the basis of guidance such as that in chapter 5, reach their own conclusions about patients' abilities to understand and contribute.

How to use the book

Because we envisage that readers may wish to dip into the book with a specific question in mind rather than read it in its entirety, each chapter is designed to be free-standing and convey as complete a picture as possible. This inevitably means that there is an overlap between chapters and repetition of some core points in each. For example, a point repeatedly emphasised throughout is the importance of children and young people being as fully involved as possible in all health care decisions

INTRODUCTION

that affect them. We also repeatedly emphasise the general desirability of shared decision making among patients, parents and health professionals while acknowledging that this is not always feasible. Chapters 2 and 3 both consider the same areas of law, pointing out where Scots law differs from the law in England, Wales and Northern Ireland. Summaries of main points are included in each chapter and the final chapter also briefly encapsulates the advice contained throughout the book. Such summaries are intended to give a quick overview but we would strongly encourage readers to consider the discussion sections rather than rely on the summaries alone.

Further advice

We have sought to flag up in the text some of the other principal sources of advice on specific subjects. In addition, information about developments following the publication of this guidance may be obtained from the BMA's website or by contacting the BMA's medical ethics department. Further details of the legal cases described can be found in published law reports, as referenced. A list of useful addresses is also provided at the end of this book.

Medical Ethics Department
British Medical Association
BMA House
Tavistock Square
London
WC1H 9JP
Tel: 020 7383 6286
Fax: 020 7383 6233
Email: ethics@bma.org.uk
Internet: www.bma.org.uk

References

1 The impact of the Human Rights Act on medical practice is discussed in Kennedy I, Grubb A. *Medical law: text with materials*, 3rd edition. London: Butterworths, 2000.
2 Human Rights Task Force. *A new era of rights and responsibilities: core guidance for public authorities*. London: Home Office, 1999.
3 *House of Lords official report (Hansard)* 1997 November 3: vol 582, col 1228.
4 Guidance for family lawyers is given in: Horowitz M, Kingscote G, Nicholls M. *The Human Rights Act 1998: a special bulletin for family lawyers*. London: Butterworths, 1999.

1: An ethical approach to treating children and young people

1.1 Focus of the book: children and young people

Attitudes to minors and to the rights accorded to them are changing. A basic aim of this book is to reflect the implications of those changing attitudes in the sphere of medical and nursing care. In all spheres of treatment, emphasis is now rightly given to listening to the views and preferences of all patients, including the young. Nevertheless, it remains the case that minors are not generally given the full range of rights and choices that they will acquire on reaching 18, the age designated as "adulthood". The reasons and possible justifications for this situation need to be re-examined and some are explored in this chapter. They centre mainly on such factors as the desire to protect the young from upsetting information and difficult decisions. While such a view is understandable, it means that children's insight and resilience have often been significantly underestimated, as have their abilities to understand and cope. Society also restricts children because of anxiety that, if given choices, they might make risky decisions that jeopardise their health. One counterargument to this is that we need, at least, to hear and understand their reasoning before assuming that it is flawed. Furthermore, as discussed below, decision making skills improve with practice, although young people should obviously not be given more responsibility than they want. Another traditional reason for limiting children's options stems from deeply rooted views about the privacy of family life and the decision making authority of parents. As is repeatedly emphasised throughout the book, in most cases of childhood illness, the whole family is deeply affected and decision making

1

is a step-by-step process to which the whole family contributes. The patient's own views must be a core part of that process, wherever possible.

As has been already mentioned in the introduction, the term "child" or "minor" generally covers everyone under the age of 18, from the newborn to the young adult. Nevertheless, even though categorised as minors, people can make some legally binding decisions prior to reaching 18. For the purposes of medical treatment, young people over the age of 16 have long been presumed competent to give consent and, if they are judged to be competent, young people under 16 can also consent to treatment independently of their parents (see chapters 2 and 3). Regarding terminology, there is a growing convention of recognising people of approximately 12 years and over as "young people", rather than "children" and this is the pattern followed loosely in this book.[1] It needs to be emphasised at the outset, however, that even if we divide minors by rough chronological age, the range of ability, awareness, insight, judgment and experience in each group is immense. Life experience and mastery of decision making skills vary considerably even within age cohorts and do not necessarily match the expectations society has about individuals' chronological age. In fact, as mentioned above, we often underestimate the abilities of children, particularly those as young as five years old and under, to understand what is at stake and, with support, to take a significant part in decisions about their health care. This is one of the problems that the book seeks to address.

1.1.1 Decision making in context

The purpose of this chapter is to consider the ethical framework within which questions of children's consent and refusal need to be considered. Although really complex ethical problems can occur in the care of children and young people, these are more the exception than the norm. Later chapters of this book discuss controversial treatments or situations in which there is a clash of opinions about treatment. Such cases are relatively rare but the same ethical concepts and established facets of good practice apply to the rare dilemmas as to the more commonly encountered situations. Very few decisions about treatment are of the life-and-death variety. Therefore, although such decisions are briefly mentioned here in order to convey the comprehensive nature of the ethical framework, they are addressed in detail only in later chapters. In all circumstances, the same basic principles about providing benefit for the patient and avoiding harm apply. In some exceptional cases, however, fine judgment is required to assess whether a particular treatment actually constitutes a benefit or might even be harmful. The views of patients themselves and their families invariably have great importance in decision making but particularly so in these finely balanced cases where doubt exists about whether a particular intervention is genuinely in the patient's best interests. Such cases raise the issue of how familiar concepts such as "best interests" and benefit and harm should be defined.

1.2 Facets of established good practice

Prioritising patients' "best interests"

A fundamental ethical obligation in the provision of treatment is that of focusing on the interests of the patient and providing benefit for that person. Competent adults are allowed to define their own concept of "best interests", even if their views about what would benefit them are very different from those of the rest of society. They can refuse treatment when they feel they have had enough or choose to take some risks with their own health. Children and young people have not generally been given the same options. Traditionally, other people — usually their parents — have chosen for them. Increasingly, however, it is being recognised that children and young people have a lot to contribute to decision making. It is also acknowledged that, although they usually coincide, the interests of the child and those of the parents are not automatically synonymous in every case. (This is discussed further below and in chapter 8.)

Regarding the definition of best interests, it is customary to assume that a person's interests are usually best served by measures that offer the hope of prolonging life or preventing damage to health. Health professionals are accustomed to measuring benefit primarily in terms of physical gains. Thus, where medical treatment carries low risk and offers substantial benefit to the patient, it is clearly perceived as being in the person's interests. This is the situation in many of the day-to-day decisions involving children although it is clear that not all choices are that simple. The side effects and other burdens of treatment may not be matched by a genuine prospect of significant and sustained improvement. Alternatively, the promise of physical improvement may necessarily involve compromises that the patient considers unacceptable, such as the administration of blood products to a Jehovah's Witness. (These more exceptional cases are discussed in chapters 2, 3 and 8.) In all cases, it is increasingly recognised that an assessment of best interests must involve far more complex matters than physical criteria alone. While not wishing to reduce such complexity to the level of a checklist, a range of general factors with social and emotional elements needs to be considered when assessing a young patient's best interests in relation to treatment.

Factors to be considered when assessing best interests:

- the patient's own ascertainable wishes, feelings and values;
- the patient's ability to understand what is proposed and weigh up the alternatives;
- the patient's potential to participate more in the decision, if provided with additional support or explanations;
- the patient's physical and emotional needs;
- the risk of harm or suffering for the patient;
- the views of parents and family;
- the implications for the family of treatment or non-treatment;
- relevant information about the patient's religious or cultural background;
- evidence of the effectiveness of the proposed treatment, particularly in relation to other options;
- the prioritising of options that maximise the patient's future opportunities and choices;
- evidence concerning the likelihood of improvement with treatment;
- evidence about the anticipated extent of improvement; and
- risks arising from delayed treatment or non-treatment.[2]

This is not intended to be an exhaustive list but it features fundamental principles that should be considered in any effort to make decisions affecting children and young people. Underlying it is the belief that children and young people are generally best cared for within the family. In some cases, they may appear uncertain of what they want to happen. Wherever possible, they must be given the time and support to assist them to make a decision with which they feel comfortable. Much of that support normally comes from the family and so emphasis should be placed on ensuring that, wherever feasible, the family is fully informed and feels involved. The significance of emotional, as well as intellectual, development in young patients must also be acknowledged.

Communication and provision of information: Good practice is based on good communication and the establishment of trust between the patient and the health team. Through every stage of their development, children should be encouraged to talk to health professionals, as well as to their families, about how they feel concerning treatment options. They should never be discouraged from asking questions about their health problems. In our view, information about their medical care should not be withheld from patients who are willing to know it, regardless of their age. We recognise that families sometimes request secrecy (particularly in the case of young patients) in order to spare the sick person from having to cope with distressing information. Health professionals can also find it difficult to be frank with patients whose prognosis is poor. In practice, however, secrecy, bad communication and the patients' suspicion that important questions are being avoided can contribute to fear and anxiety. Research shows that children benefit from knowing about important factors in their parents' health, and from being given truthful explanations.[3] Dishonesty undermines trust and can create a barrier between patients and health professionals.

Listening to the child: It is essential that children and young people are shown that their views are valued and, where appropriate, that those views will be treated confidentially, on the same terms as dialogue with other patients. (Chapter 4 considers both the scope and limitations of the duty of confidentiality.) In fact, the ethics of providing care and treatment for minors are the same in most respects as the ethics of treating any other patient. Young patients are individuals whose interests need to be considered in a broad manner that takes account of their physical needs, their own wishes and the circumstances of the case.

Encouraging development of decision making skills: It is generally accepted that, as young people mature, they increasingly take a larger degree of the responsibility for decisions that closely affect them. As we discuss in chapter 5, the ethical duties of health professionals include the obligation to enhance their patients' competence and ability to participate, where it is possible to do so, by measures such as explaining the options in an accessible way and in familiar surroundings. The health team has a duty to ensure that the patient's contribution is not overlooked and that he or she has the information necessary to form a view. Children and young people acquire the skills to make sound and reasoned decisions by having opportunities to weigh up the options and exercise choices. The former Master of the Rolls, Lord Donaldson, has said, for example, that:

> *Adolescence is a period of progressive transition from childhood to adulthood and as experience of life is acquired and intelligence and understanding grow, so will the scope of the decision-making which should be left to the minor, for it is only by making decisions and experiencing the consequences that decision-making skills will be acquired ... good parenting involves giving minors as much rope as they can handle without an unacceptable risk that they will hang themselves.*[4]

Provision of support: It is axiomatic that care should focus on the best interests of the patient. In the case of children and young people, those interests are generally intertwined with those of their close relatives. Children and young people generally live in networks of emotional relationships that are important to them. Usually, the interests of the young patient and the family coincide.[5] Both in routine care and in exceptional dilemmas, health professionals weigh up medical factors, the patient's wishes and those of the family. Parents generally know the child better than anyone else and are best placed to assess the child's interests and support the child emotionally through the illness. In cases of serious disease, the whole family is also likely to need advice and support from the health team. In most cases, a close dialogue between parents and the health team is the best way of deciding on treatment options for young, immature children. Parents should also be closely involved in decision making with mature children, wherever this is consistent with the principle of confidentiality.

Confidentiality: All patients are entitled to privacy and confidentiality. Nevertheless, situations arise where patients of any age should be encouraged to share information with other people who are closely affected by it. Children and young people should be particularly encouraged to do so and to involve their parents in decision making. The kinds of situations in which they may refuse to do so are discussed in chapter 8, which includes advice on provision of contraception, abortion and treatment for sexually transmitted diseases. Despite the presumption of a right to confidentiality in most situations, circumstances can arise for patients of any age in which secrecy cannot be maintained because of the risks involved. Evidence of abuse, neglect or exploitation of children or young people requires health professionals to take action (see chapter 4 and appendix 1). Wherever possible, the first step must be to talk to the child or young person concerned in an attempt to gain his or her permission to pass information to an appropriate authority and to ensure that the patient's trust in health professionals is not undermined.

1.2.1 Summary of good practice

Some established principles define the manner in which treatment of children and young people should be approached.

- Children and young people should be kept as fully informed as they wish and as is possible about their care and treatment. They also have a right to exempt themselves from all or some aspects of decision making about their treatment although, wherever possible, they should be encouraged to make their general preferences known.
- The wishes and values of children and young people should always be taken into account. The individual's overall welfare should be the paramount consideration and listening to patients is conducive to promoting their welfare in the widest sense.
- The multifaceted needs, including emotional needs, of children should be recognised.
- Children and young people should be encouraged to make all those decisions that they feel comfortable, and able, to make. In the majority of cases, young people who have an understanding of what is involved can make responsible and reasoned decisions about medical treatment options.

- Although minors should be treated in such a way as to promote their personal responsibility consistent with their needs, they should also be encouraged to take decisions in collaboration with other family members, especially parents, if this is feasible.
- Wherever possible, decision making should not be hurried. Patients and families often need time to reflect and talk. Health professionals can help by providing as much evidence-based information as possible and being willing to discuss the options in a supportive environment.

1.3 Recognising minors' rights

Ideally, the provision of appropriate health care should be a matter of common agreement between patients, people close to them and the health team. Discussion of the rights of various parties can appear confrontational in such a context. Nevertheless, many commentators predict an increased focus on rights in health care as a result of factors such as the generally growing emphasis on patient and consumer choice and changes in practice reflecting the Human Rights Act 1998. (Some legal as well as ethical issues are mentioned in this section but the law is discussed in more detail in chapters 2 and 3.)

1.3.1 Minors' rights in the context of parental autonomy

Legal experts point out that, in law, the Human Rights Act "marks a radical change of approach to traditional thinking on how best to protect the rights and freedoms of British citizens".[6] Nevertheless, as the Act at the time of writing is only recently enacted, the extent to which children are likely to benefit directly from it remains unclear, although it is expected that all patient groups will benefit in the long term from the increasing awareness of rights generally. In Fortin's view children "will inevitably benefit from the heightened rights consciousness"[7] but she also reminds us that they are not the key focus of the Act. Minors have rights under the Human Rights Act just like everyone else but, as for everyone else, their rights will have to be interpreted in relation to the rights of other people. In legal cases involving children, the rights and authority of parents are also likely to be considered. This is because embodied in the Act are Articles of the European Convention on Human Rights, which takes a broad approach to rights, focused on the rights of individuals in relation to the state authorities.[8] The specific rights of children are not central here because most children live in a family setting, and "adult carers stand interposed between them and the state".[9] Fortin goes on to say that, from a children's perspective, a potential problem with the European Convention and the case law arising from it is the implicit assumption that parents' rights are likely to be identical with their children's rights. She notes that:

[T]he Articles and Convention case law reinforce the common view advocated by most legal systems throughout the world that the value of family life lies in its privacy from state interference; furthermore, that family privacy involves parental autonomy.[10]

Nevertheless, perceptions of parental authority are subtly changing, influenced by such factors as the growing number of families extended by step-parents, half-siblings and children who commute between two parental homes. Notions of family privacy are also challenged by increasing societal awareness of issues such as domestic violence and child abuse. As is discussed in later chapters, the law is changing to accommodate trends such as that of unmarried parenthood by re-examining the legal issue of parental responsibility and, in case law, by insisting that consent from one parent alone is insufficient for non-therapeutic interventions such as male infant circumcision (see section 6.1.1). In our view, while uncertainty remains regarding the extent to which practice will change in relation to minors' rights as a result of the Human Rights Act, such rights are increasingly seen as an important matter for debate and re-evaluation. Indeed, this is demonstrated by the factors that have given rise to this book. The fact that health professionals continue to express uncertainty about the rights of minors to consent or refuse medical treatment independently of their parents indicates that parental authority is far from clear in all cases. It is conceivable, therefore, that as we become more accustomed to looking at a range of issues, such as health care, through the prism of human rights, views about parental authority over competent children will also undergo significant change.

In everyday practice, health professionals have long been

accustomed to striving to balance the potentially conflicting needs and wishes of the individual young person and that of his or her family. They do so by acknowledging their own ethical duties to ensure the best interests of the patient and by being willing to speak out when the parents' views appear inconsistent with the patient's interests. Good practice also takes practical considerations into account, including factors such as the difficulties inherent in attempting to force treatment and compliance with aftercare on an unwilling patient who feels excluded from the decision making process that led to that treatment and aftercare.

1.3.2 Ethical and practical considerations

An inherent problem in statements of rights is the lack of any widely agreed way of ranking different rights that may not sit easily with one another, and of balancing one person's rights with those of other people, for instance with those of parents and siblings. Much discussion of the Human Rights Act focuses on concepts such as proportionality and legitimate aims, emphasising that the rights of individuals have to be interpreted within a framework that takes account of other factors. Similar considerations come into play when looking at rights and duties from an ethical perspective. As well as ensuring that individuals' rights are respected, medical ethics is also concerned with balance and ensuring, for example, that benefits are not pursued at the cost of significant harm, either to the young patient or to other people. All patients have the right to say what should or should not be done to them but most rights are not absolute and have to be in proportion with other values that society considers important.

Competent children and young people: Health professionals should act as the patient's advocate whenever it seems that his or her views are not fully represented within the decision making process. In practice, it is often hard to make a rigid distinction between the best interests of the patient and those of the family. The whole family's emotional and psychological welfare is likely to be intimately linked to the child's prognosis and, similarly, the child's sense of wellbeing may be affected by the family's attitude. There is now consensus that from a young age children ought to be consulted and involved in health care choices.[11] This does not necessarily mean they should be the sole decision makers or be able automatically to overrule the views of people caring for them. Children's and young people's ability to grasp what is involved in the treatment choice is the principal criterion as to whether or not their views have a major effect on that decision. (Assessment of competence is discussed in chapter 5.)

Children and young people who lack competence: Even when they do not fully understand, minors still have a right to be told what they want to know about their health care and helped to express their views about that. Adults should make genuine efforts to accommodate the child's preferences, where possible. This needs to be done, however, within a treatment plan that takes account of the particular needs and wishes of the patient and of the family. In practice, serious decisions for patients of any age are seldom made in strict isolation but with the support of other people, such as friends, partners, families, carers and health professionals. Adults choose whom they wish to involve in the decision and mature children can also generally claim this right. For young children, unless there is evidence to the contrary, the expectation is that parents are the appropriate primary decision makers. In the vast majority of cases, they know the child better than anyone and are the best judge of where the child's best interests lie.

UN Convention on the Rights of the Child: Internationally, the UN's 1989 Convention on the Rights of the Child is the most widely endorsed statement of children's rights and, in contrast with the European Convention on Human Rights mentioned above, children and young people are its focus of concern.[12] In 1991, the UK ratified the UN Convention, accepting responsibility for the development of rights-based and child-centred health care. The Convention sets out standards that should be reflected in the health care sphere and in other areas. They are consistent with the UK's domestic laws about children.[13] Article 3 of the UN Convention states that any decision or action affecting children and young people, either as individuals or as a group, should be focused on their best interests (see section 1.2 above).

The UN Convention also imposes responsibilities on the state and on parents and guardians to ensure that all children are properly looked after, educated and provided with good quality health care. The state has obligations to enact legislation and implement all measures necessary to ensure that the rights set out in the UN Convention are put into practice. Parents and carers have the main responsibility for bringing up and protecting children but they, in turn, are entitled to support, advice and services in order to fulfil these obligations. A child has a right under the Convention not to be separated from his or her parents or carers unless it is judged to be in the child's best interests.

1.3.3 Why assessment of minors' rights can be complex

Discussion of children's rights is complex because much of the normal focus on patient rights is directed at issues of choice, autonomy and self-determination. Health professionals have come to associate the notion of patient rights with the legally binding power of adult patients to refuse or limit certain treatments. Competent adult patients have very strong rights in respect of accepting or refusing treatment and, logically, the closer a young person is to achieving similar competence, the more the moral weight should shift towards prioritising that person's right of self-determination. In practice, however, the situation with regard to minors' rights seldom seems that straightforward. Although competent children's right to self-determination is much debated, in practice it is usually limited if their health would be seriously jeopardised as a result of their choices. This is one respect in which the treatment of minors differs significantly from that of adults, where patient autonomy allows for treatment refusal even when death results. Society has an interest in ensuring that young people's health is not avoidably put at risk.

Assessment of young people's rights is in many ways more complex than debate about the rights of adults partly because societal attitudes to minors are somewhat ambivalent. For children and young people, the courts provide an ultimate arbiter. In England, Wales and Northern Ireland, they can override a child's refusal or parents' proxy refusal of a particular treatment if there is evidence that it would provide significant benefit (see chapters 2, 3 and 6). It is not the aim of this book to argue that society or the courts should countenance more risk-taking in relation to children's health but rather to draw attention to some of the ambiguities that health professionals face in meeting society's expectations. In terms of patient rights, health professionals are encouraged both to respect young people's wishes and to protect them by ensuring their right to good health care.

1.3.4 Equity, non-discrimination and other important rights

It is important to recognise that autonomy and self-determination are not the only ethical considerations, or even necessarily the most important rights, for children. Among the rights particularly mentioned in the UN Convention, for example, are those of children with disabilities who have the right to assistance in order to achieve social integration and individual development. In the past, health organisations and patient groups have called attention to discriminative practices that effectively exclude some children, especially those with disabilities, from even being considered for some forms of life-prolonging medical treatment. Transparent and equitable procedures whereby such patients can be individually considered for treatment need to be in place. Blanket decision making that appears to disadvantage some patients or discriminate between patients on grounds other than clinical need is ethically unacceptable and may be unlawful under the Human Rights Act.

In 1995, the former British Paediatric Association, now the Royal College of Paediatrics and Child Health (RCPCH), published a paediatrician's brief guide to the UN Convention, welcoming the opportunity for paediatricians and other health professionals to work towards a paradigm shift within society on the matter of children's health care rights.[14] The guide focuses on, for instance, the right of competent children to make informed choices and the right of confidentiality. It highlights Article 12 of the UN Convention, which obliges health professionals to seek the opinion of children and young people before taking decisions that affect them. It emphasises that children should be informed of the nature of the treatment and be involved in choices about alternatives. The RCPCH sees these rights as "particularly important in children with chronic illnesses such as cystic fibrosis, diabetes, cancer or renal failure". More generally, the guidance also addresses the child's right to "the enjoyment of the highest attainable standard of health". It points out that this basic right has been breached by widening inequalities in child health, with poverty and deprivation contributing significantly to the risks of infant and childhood mortality and morbidity.[15] The College calls upon doctors to help identify children at highest risk of suboptimal health, including those whose families are on low incomes or affected by homelessness. Recognising the increasing numbers of young refugees and asylum seekers in Britain, including increasing numbers of unaccompanied minors applying for asylum, the need for equity of access to health services for cultural and ethnic minorities and disadvantaged families has also been highlighted. The right to consent to and refuse treatment — which is our basic concern in this book — must be seen within a wider framework of rights that respect children as whole individuals.

1.3.5 Health workers as patient advocates

Various organisations have highlighted the particular relevance for health workers of the rights set out in the UN Convention. The British Association for Community Child Health, in association with other organisations, has published a detailed practitioners' guide that sets out checklists for the implementation in health care of the rights embodied in the UN Convention.[16] The guide particularly emphasises the duty of health professionals to act as advocates and to provide children and young people with information about their rights in the health sphere. The health care rights of children and young people are also set out in advisory statements such as the World Medical Association's Declaration on the Rights of the Child to Health Care.[17] This statement also gives general recognition to a range of minors' rights, including the rights to care and protection and freedom of choice.

1.3.6 Summary of minors' basic health rights

Children have rights
- to child-centred health care;
- to be looked after appropriately, without discrimination of any kind including on grounds of disability;
- to be encouraged in every way possible to develop their full potential;
- to take opportunities to be involved, from the beginning, and to choose not to be involved in decision making;
- to receive clear information about matters closely affecting themselves and about the right to decline detailed information at a particular time;
- to have opportunities to express opinions without pressure or criticism;
- to receive support and encouragement in decision making;
- to ask someone else to decide a particular issue;

- to receive an explanation of the reasons when their preference cannot be met;
- to confidentiality; and
- to redress — where appropriate — through a fast, accessible complaints procedure.

1.4 Consent to and refusal of medical treatment

At the heart of this book is a question concerning the extent to which children and young people can consent to or refuse treatment independently of the views of other people. In this section the focus is primarily on *ethical* and *practical* aspects of consent and refusal. (The *law* on consent is explained in chapters 2 and 3.)

Consent: From an ethical perspective, any informed and competent patient can authorise a medical procedure, once the implications, side effects and alternatives have been appropriately explained. Age is not necessarily a major factor for valid consent. Nevertheless, in practice, it is generally prudent to obtain the consent of parents (or people with parental responsibility) for any serious or risky intervention for children and for those whose level of understanding is in doubt. Clearly, parents can authorise or refuse treatment on behalf of babies and young children in accordance with their best interests. Even with older children and young people who consent to treatment, it is desirable in most situations to have parental consent in addition to the patient's own, so that the family is able to support the young person in making the treatment decision. Nevertheless, on sensitive matters such as obtaining family planning advice, termination of pregnancy, treatment of sexually transmitted diseases or addiction, young people are frequently reluctant to allow parents to be informed, despite encouragement from health professionals to do so (see also chapter 8). In these cases, as long as health professionals feel confident that the patient is able to make an informed decision to authorise treatment and the benefits of involving parents have been discussed, treatment can proceed on the young person's authorisation.

Consent can be verbal, written or signalled by the acquiescence of a person who understands what will be undertaken. Absence of refusal, however expressed, may therefore constitute consent as long as the person understands the procedure to be undertaken and its implications and is aware that rejecting it is an available option. Acquiescence when the person does not know what the intervention entails or that there is an option of refusing it is not "consent". Nor is a mere signature on a consent form proof of valid consent. The importance accorded to the signature is entirely dependent upon the quality of the information that has been provided and the recipient's understanding of that information.

Refusal: Refusal of treatment by a child or young person who properly understands the implications is an ethically important consideration and should be taken very seriously even though in some circumstances the law may permit parents and the courts to overrule such a refusal (see sections 2.2.1 and 3.2.4). At any age, a patient who has already experienced and remembers the treatment in question is better equipped to assess it than a patient who has not. The better informed the patient is, the more convincing his or her decision will appear. Furthermore, where families support the young patient's view, this adds substantially to its weight and authority.

Valid and invalid refusal: Children sometimes refuse treatment because their anxieties are focused on one aspect of it that may not be the most important element, for example, the short term fear of an injection that is necessary before a bigger procedure, such as surgery. They are not expressing a considered choice in favour of non-treatment and they might willingly accept the intervention if administered differently, for example if they were given anaesthetising cream before the injection. Genuine refusal of treatment is based on awareness of the implications, is consistent over time and is compatible with the child's view of his or her best interests beyond the short term. In cases where non-treatment will necessarily result in grave harm, suffering or death, society requires the patient to have a full understanding of all the implications and details. Where the refusal appears consistent, valid and informed but would be likely to result in serious and avoidable damage to the patient's health, legal advice should be sought.

The understanding required for valid refusal: The degree of understanding required for any decision must be commensurate with the gravity of the matter being decided. For instance, a greater degree of understanding may be required to refuse a potentially life-prolonging therapy than that required to consent to it, since the implications of refusal are likely to be more serious. There are, however, exceptions: sometimes consenting may require even more understanding than declining. Consenting to a risky procedure may be just as hazardous as refusing an innovative therapy whose full effects may be unpredictable (see also section 9.6). Outside the sphere of life-prolonging treatment, an example of treatment for which consent requires a very high degree of understanding is surgery for gender reassignment. Where young people desire such treatment, they would be expected to demonstrate a very thorough awareness of the implications for their whole lives.

1.4.1 Why we value patient consent

Modern medical ethics sets great value on self-determination and respect for patient choice. Individuals are encouraged to take responsibility for their own welfare by, for example, receiving information that will help them prevent illness. It is desirable for patients of all ages and abilities to have a voice in decisions about their health and to be able to exercise as much control as possible about what is done to their bodies. Health professionals have a duty to take all reasonable steps to enhance patients' abilities to do this. Law and ethics also require that treatment of children and young people be based on an assessment of their best interests. As mentioned above, in the past this was often interpreted only in terms of striving for measurable clinical improvement, regardless of the patient's priorities, but it is now recognised that a strong element of any person's best interests is that the person's own choices and preferences are respected.

In the case of serious illness or disability, consent usually involves a series of decisions. It has a practical importance. Compliance with a treatment regime is more likely when patients accept it, understand the reason for it and take responsibility for maintaining their health. In many areas of treatment, compliance with a long term regime of health care is essential to its success.

1.4.2 When can patients refuse treatment?

Clearly, real choice involves the option of making what might be perceived as bad decisions as well as allowing people to choose options that others consider to be unwise.

Adults are acknowledged to have very clear rights to make unwise decisions. They can choose, within the limits of what they are offered, things that will foreseeably harm or disadvantage them. As long as they are mentally competent, the only limits on adults' choices are the duties to act within the law and to not damage others. Only if there is evidence that adults suffer from impairment to their judgment or mental faculties do others feel justified in intervening without their consent. So, when an adult patient makes a medical decision that appears conducive to self harm, the issues upon which health professionals must satisfy themselves are whether the decision is within the law, whether it harms other people, whether that person has sufficient mental competence to make the particular decision and whether enough information about it has been provided. This is also the starting point for decision making by children and young people under the age of majority.

Children and young people face a more complicated situation than people over 18 who can refuse treatment for reasons that are good, bad or for no reason at all. In England, Wales and Northern Ireland, minors do not have unlimited rights to refuse treatment. A refusal is most likely to be respected when the young patient clearly understands the nature and implications of the particular intervention and the treatment is not seen as crucial to his or her welfare at that time (assessment of the validity of refusal is discussed in section 6.1.2). This means that there is a sliding scale of measures that children and young people may be able to refuse. A minor's informed and competent refusal of an elective or non-urgent treatment should generally be respected unless there are some exceptional arguments to the contrary, such as a risk of damage in the long term or harm to other people. Health professionals are always extremely reluctant to enforce treatment unless it is essential to do so to save life or prevent a serious deterioration in health. As implied previously, to overrule an individual's valid wishes without the strongest justification cannot be considered as acting in the patient's interests. Thus, the medical procedures that are least essential to their wellbeing are generally the most amenable to an informed refusal. Where the law permits, those that are immediately life-prolonging or essential to maintain the young patient's health are least likely to be withheld, simply on the basis of the child's refusal. In the latter case, questions arise about the child's competence and moral authority to make such a grave decision. Ultimately, the matter may need to be referred to the courts (see sections 2.5.3 and 3.5.3). Ideally, however, medical decisions are best made in partnership by the patient, the family and the health team. The parental role as primary decision maker gradually fades as the child develops in maturity, although the importance of parents as a source of emotional support and advice should, ideally, remain. The limits on the rights of parents to refuse are discussed in sections 2.3.2, 3.3.2 and 6.1.1.

1.4.3 Why are mature children and young people treated differently from adults?

Discussions about minors' consent to medical treatment tend to be dominated by the twin issues of whether they are competent to make informed decisions and whether, even if they are competent, it is right to allow them to make serious and difficult choices.[18] In fact, society at large can be said to wish to promote mutually incompatible values when it emphasises the right of informed and mature young people to make autonomous decisions but, at the same time, insists on protecting them from the effects of those decisions. Society often adds an additional hurdle for children and young people who wish to decide for themselves. As well as demonstrating their competence to understand the implications of the choice, they must also reassure those around them that they can make the "right" choice. In practice, this has tended to mean that their views are only likely to be implemented when they conform to other people's notion of their welfare. That is to say, young patients have often been given an opportunity to consent to whatever medical treatment is offered to them but not to refuse it when it is recommended.

Increasingly, however, health professionals are unwilling to override what might be perceived as an unwise decision by a young person, particularly if the patient appears to have weighed up the arguments carefully or has prior experience of the particular treatment on offer. The BMA sees evidence of doctors increasingly doubting their authority to proceed where a young person refuses and looking to the courts for guidance (see chapters 2 and 3). In practical terms, doctors are also often worried about ensuring willing compliance with aftercare if the patient has been an unwilling recipient of treatment.

AN ETHICAL APPROACH TO TREATING

1.4.4 Exceptionally grave decisions

Treatment choices that have extremely grave adverse implications are exceptional and are invariably challenging to any person. Nevertheless, the same ethical principles to do with establishing trust, providing information and listening to patients' views apply equally here as elsewhere. A child or young person who has already experienced serious illness and various forms of medical treatment may be as well equipped as an older person to decide whether to agree to further similar treatment. Very hard choices arise when serious disability or death is an inevitable consequence of the disease and treatment only offers a slender hope of benefit. Whatever their age, patients' own preferences should carry much weight in these circumstances. This is clearly not the same, however, as saying that society should accept unquestioningly a non-treatment decision by a child or young person whose medical condition appears amenable to successful treatment. Part of the difficulty with acknowledging that children and young people often have sufficient competence to make valid choices in important as well as trivial matters is that society generally wishes both to empower and to protect young people. These two aims can be incompatible and when they conflict, this creates particular dilemmas for health professionals.

Although confrontation clearly needs to be avoided and, wherever possible agreement should be reached through dialogue and negotiation with young patients, this is not always possible. The courts are then brought in to arbitrate and ensure that decisions are made with transparency and due consideration of all pertinent factors. Although this chapter is primarily about ethics and moral values, we need to mention briefly the role of the judiciary since the courts can be seen as representing societal moral priorities. As mentioned earlier in the chapter, although treatment decisions are primarily matters for the patient, family and health team, the wider community also has responsibilities to ensure that children are properly cared for. Society's concerns are reflected in court proceedings and media debate. The courts base judgments on a balancing of the risks of overriding the young person's apparent wishes against other risks, such as serious damage to health or death. Debate about this matter came to the fore in a 1999 High Court judgment that sought to reconcile apparently incompatible societal aims: to follow a young person's expressed wishes, or save her life against her will.[19]

M's refusal of a heart transplant

M was a 15-year-old who refused to consent to a heart transplant operation in 1999 when her own heart failed. Her mother gave legal consent on her behalf but health professionals were unwilling to proceed without M's agreement. M said she did not want to die but neither did she wish to have the transplant since this would make her feel different from other people. "I understand what a heart transplant means, procedure explained ... checkups ... tablets for the rest of your life. I feel depressed about that. I am only fifteen and don't want to take tablets for the rest of my life ... I don't want to die. It's hard to take it all in ... If I had children ... I would not let them die ... I don't want to die, but I would rather die than have the transplant ... I would feel different with someone else's heart, that's a good enough reason not to have a heart transplant, even if it saved my life".[20] After listening to her views, Mr Justice Johnson decided that M was not capable of making the decision herself and he authorised the operation to go ahead despite her reluctance. "Events have overtaken her so swiftly that she has not been able to come to terms with her situation",[21] he said. Once that decision had been made on her behalf, M agreed to comply with treatment.

Re M (Child: Refusal of Medical Treatment)

As in other similar cases, the judge emphasised that, normally, young people's best interests lie in having their integrity respected and their decisions on personal matters supported. Nevertheless, he said, there might come a point where the powers that society invests in the legal system would be meaningless if there were no valid means of overriding a young person's decision to refuse life-saving treatment. He recognised the risks of the patient carrying resentment for her whole life about the decision made on her behalf. He said that this risk, however, was impossible to assess accurately and had to be weighed against not just a risk but the certainty of her death, if action were not taken. In discussing the law and other legal precedents, however, the judge focused on the moral arguments. He quoted Lord Justice Balcombe in a previous case, who maintained that:

Undoubtedly, the philosophy ... is that, as children approach the age of majority, they are increasingly able to take their own decisions concerning their medical treatment. In logic there can be no difference between an ability to consent to treatment and an ability to refuse treatment ... Accordingly the older the child concerned the greater the weight the court should give to its wishes, certainly in the field of medical treatment. In a sense this is merely one aspect of the application of the test that the welfare of the child is the paramount consideration.[22]

1.4.5 The welfare of the child

Where the child is too young and immature to make a valid decision, parents are the normal arbiters of where a child's best interests lie and how the child's welfare can be promoted. Society, however, is ready to intervene if parents appear to make unwise decisions for their children, even though it would not stop parents making similar decisions for themselves. The moral justification is that society has special obligations to protect its most vulnerable members, among whom are children and young people. As we have seen earlier in the chapter, this is also one of the moral responsibilities that governments accept in ratifying the UN Convention on the Rights of the Child. The following case about testing a young baby for HIV is also discussed in sections 2.3.2 and 3.3.2.[23]

The welfare of child C

C was almost five months old in September 1999 when the local authority applied to the High Court to allow a blood test to be taken to ascertain C's HIV status. Her parents were vehemently opposed to a blood test. C's mother had tested HIV positive in 1990 and again in 1998 but remained in good health and symptom-free. Both parents were very sceptical about the conventional medical approach to HIV. C's mother had, therefore, rejected medical advice about avoidance of mother-to-baby HIV transmission during pregnancy and labour. She refused a Caesarean section, opted to breast-feed and rejected the GP's advice that C should be tested and, if positive, be given prophylactic medication. The judge heard that C was at about 15% risk of infection during pregnancy and birth and that breast-feeding increased the risk by between 5% and 10%. C's mother said she intended to breast-feed until C reached the age of 18 months or 2 years. Medical experts advised that this

---

increased the risks of transmission by 3% each year.

Mr Justice Wilson acknowledged the importance of parental views and said that these must feature in the overarching enquiry into C's welfare. He considered whether, in general, the united wishes of both parents should be perceived as correctly identifying a child's welfare and suggested this should be a rebuttable presumption. Nevertheless, he said that on the evidence provided in this instance, the parents' plans for protecting the child amounted to a "hopeless programme". He concluded that baby C had rights of her own that could not be subsumed within the rights of parents. The judge quoted various provisions of the UN Convention on the Rights of the Child, including the duty of the state to "ensure to the maximum extent possible the survival and development of the child"[24] and "the right of the child to the enjoyment of the highest attainable standard of health".[25] The court, therefore, ordered that testing take place.

Re C (A child) (HIV testing)

1.5 Criteria for valid decision making

In order for their decisions to carry moral weight, children and young people must be seen as capable of exercising judgment on the particular issue that requires a decision. Several fundamental criteria must be satisfied in order for any person to be deemed capable of decision making. The criteria vary according to the decision to be made but basically require a person to have relevant information about all the options plus an appropriate level of understanding and experience (see also chapter 5). Clearly, choosing between several options that are likely to have roughly equivalent outcomes differs from trying to weigh up the merits of options with vastly different consequences. It is also likely that competence to choose which school to attend or which examinations to take requires a child to have different skills from being able to decide about medical treatment.[26] Within medicine, there are profound variations in the gravity of the decisions to be made.

Children are clearly able to decide upon some aspects of treatment without necessarily being competent to determine every issue. To take a simple example, choosing between having an injection in one's left or right arm requires a much lower level of understanding and experience than choosing not to have it at all, since the latter choice may have serious consequences. In children, as in adults, competence can only be judged in relation to the particular decision that is at stake. It requires an awareness of the fact that choices have consequences and that different and specific implications arise from each choice. While perhaps complicated to describe, most people recognise what is involved in expressing preferences and feel able to do so on a range of issues from an early age.

As previously discussed, a significant difference between children and adults is that people over 16 are presumed competent to make any decision, no matter how complex, until it is proved otherwise. For younger people the reverse is seen as the norm in that they are often perceived as incapable of forming reasoned views on any important issue. In our view, this anomaly needs to be addressed and this book seeks to encourage a rethink and more debate about such assumptions. Excluding babies and the very young, children and young people are generally competent to have a coherent view on a wide range of matters. Some of these matters they can decide for themselves as long as they understand what the choice involves and its foreseeable implications. Clearly, they also need information about the consequences of the alternative options in a readily understandable form. In addition, it is increasingly recognised that for all patients, decisions are based, not only on an understanding of the issues, but on a range of factors, including intuition and emotion. We support the suggestion that "a more realistic and respectful understanding of reason, instead of seeing it as clouded and distorted by emotion, is to see that feeling, memory and imagination can be sources of great insight".[27]

1.5.1 Weighing "benefits" and "burdens"

Exceptional though they may be, particularly difficult human and ethical dilemmas arise when seriously ill people refuse potentially life-prolonging treatment or request interventions which health professionals do not think will genuinely improve their condition. The core purpose of medicine is to provide benefit for patients, whatever their age and circumstances. But assessing "benefit" increasingly involves complex and conflicting arguments. As we have already made clear, having one's own values respected by other people is clearly a benefit and, in some circumstances, society values this above the benefit of keeping the person alive. Thus, adults are not given treatment against their wishes even though this would clearly save lives; the risks of forcibly inflicting treatment are recognised as so great as to make medical treatment a harm rather than a benefit.

Such dilemmas are greatly exacerbated when the patient is a child or young person. There is some evidence that implies that health care decisions are approached differently for this population than for adult patients. Research indicates, for example, that health professionals tend to want to treat children and young people even in circumstances where they would not generally offer prolongation of treatment to an adult with the same condition. Doctors "frequently give young patients more chances to revive from and survive their illnesses than they offer to older, particularly elderly patients. Clinicians also seem more willing to impose greater burdens on children with fewer chances of success than on adults".[28] Part of this difference in attitude may be attributable to the fact that outcomes can be less predictable in children than in older patients but it also is indicative of health professionals wanting to give young people every chance of survival, even against the odds. The death of a child is universally seen as one of the most tragic experiences but, equally, there is a clear awareness that futile and invasive overtreatment must be avoided. Although we repeatedly emphasise that disputes on life and death issues are highly exceptional, unfortunately they can occur and, in such cases, legal advice should be sought.

1.6 Involving minors in health care decisions

Throughout this chapter, emphasis is placed on the fundamental ethical principle that all patients who have some mental capacity, regardless of their age, should be properly informed in a way they can understand about medical matters that pertain to them (see also section 5.4.1). They must have the opportunity to be involved as much as they are able and willing to be, in all aspects of decision making about their care and treatment. In cases where these principles are not followed, the onus must be on health professionals to demonstrate that either giving information would be inappropriate or that the patient does not want to make decisions.

Such justification could arise when individuals' level of understanding is demonstrably so extremely limited that it is impossible to discuss the issues with them. If there is evidence that it would be damaging to involve them in decision making or where patients are clearly reluctant to know the details, information should not be forced upon them. A key issue concerns the way in which health professionals assess an individual child's level of understanding and his or her ability to engage in meaningful dialogue about medical matters. At this point, it is sufficient to note that studies of young children's conversations make clear that pre-schoolers as young as three and four years of age can discuss issues and engage in decision making.[29] Obviously, the ways in which they do so, and their capacity to deal with complex matters, varies.

Earlier in the chapter it was argued that people learn how to make decisions by practice and by having the opportunity to exercise decision making skills (see section 1.2). People learn by experience from their mistakes. Therefore, society needs to allow children and young people to make some errors. Nevertheless, society requires there to be a safety net to ensure that the risks taken are confined within widely agreed parameters and therefore, in some circumstances, children's choices may be overridden when the risks of implementing them appear excessive.

1.6.1 When should minors be protected from decision making?

A valid reason for withholding information or leaving people out of decision making is that it would be harmful to them to do otherwise. In the past, it was usual for doctors to "protect" adult patients from worry by withholding difficult information from them or by being misleadingly optimistic. Such paternalism is no longer acceptable. Medical ethics requires that health professionals discuss diagnoses, prognoses and treatment options honestly with patients. If young people are deprived of the facts necessary to inform their choice, the law is unlikely to judge them to be competent to make the decision (see section 5.4.1). Opportunities for information sharing should be made available, while recognising that there are valid individual differences in the extent to which patients wish to be involved in the detail. Above all, prevarication and deliberate misinformation should be avoided. Questions should be answered sensitively but honestly.

Thus, at least after the early pre-school years, it is never acceptable for children to be excluded totally from participating in decision making on matters of health care that concern them. The weight given to their views should properly be influenced by the level of their understanding. This does not necessarily mean that children, or even young adolescents, should be expected to be the final arbiter when the decision is a serious one. They are used to turning to parents for advice and guidance and many young people continue to do so on serious matters throughout their adolescence.[30]

Just as all patients have a right to be informed about aspects of their own health, so they usually also have the opportunity to choose not to have detailed information. While valid decisions cannot be made without information, children or adult patients may want to exempt themselves from decision making that seems too difficult or emotionally painful and may ask someone else to decide for them. Sometimes the decision not to be informed is a temporary one that gives the individual a breathing space to adjust. Therefore, information should always be on offer and patients should be aware that they can change their minds and opt back into a decision making role. Parents may also desire to protect children from bad news. Although health professionals need to pay attention to what families say about patients' sensitivities, feelings and wishes, nevertheless, the starting point has to be the right of all individuals to be properly informed and to be able to participate in decision making as much as they are able to do so.

Shared decision making is the preferred option in most instances. Perhaps the most obvious circumstance when it is particularly damaging to force (or expect) children to take the final decision is when one parent argues for one course and the other parent presses for the opposite. Inevitably, such decisions will be felt by the child as having an element of conflict over loyalty. Ordinarily, children are not, and should not, be expected to choose between their parents and such cases require sensitive management so that the child feels empowered to indicate his or her own preferences.

1.7 Summary

- Children and young people should be given information about their health in ways they can readily understand. While distressing information should never be forced on patients, their questions should be answered as truthfully and sensitively as possible.
- In most cases, parents are the best judges of what is best for babies and very young children. Parental support is also important for older children and young people and the latter should be encouraged to involve their parents in health care decisions.
- Children are constantly developing. As their experience and maturity grows, children should play an ever greater role in decisions.
- Whereas it may seem logical for children and young people to have just as much opportunity to refuse as to consent to treatment, in practice their options to decline procedures recommended for them are generally limited. In the face of a young patient's apparently competent, informed and valid refusal of an essential treatment, legal advice should be sought.
- In relation to elective treatments or circumstances in which the treatment may be recommended but lacks any urgency, a young person's valid refusal should carry great weight. In practice in such cases, health professionals would not wish to see treatment enforced unless the reasons for it were urgent and compelling.

References

1 This is the convention adopted in, for example: Ministry of Health, New Zealand. *Consent in child and youth health: information for practitioners.* Wellington: Ministry of Health, 1998.
2 Based on an extract from British Medical Association. *Consent toolkit.* London: BMA, in press.
3 Barnes J, Kroll L, Burke O, Lee J, Jones A, Stein A. Qualitative interview study of communication between parents and children about maternal breast cancer. *BMJ* 2000;**321**:479—82.
4 Former Master of the Rolls, Lord Donaldson in Re W (A Minor) (Medical Treatment: Court's Jurisdiction) [1993] Fam 64 at 81F-G, [1992] 3 WLR 758, [1992] 4 All ER 627 at 638, CA.
5 Circumstances in which this is not the case, such as when young people wish to withhold information from their parents or when parents want children to undergo controversial treatment such as organ donation, are considered in later chapters.
6 Fortin J. Rights brought home for children. *The Modern Law Review* 1999;**62**:350—70:350.
7 Fortin J. Rights brought home for children. *The Modern Law Review* 1999;**62**:350—70:352.

8 Convention for the Protection of Human Rights and Fundamental Freedoms (4. ix. 1950; TS 71; Cmnd 8969).
9 Fortin J. Rights brought home for children. *The Modern Law Review* 1999;**62**:350—70:355.
10 Fortin J. Rights brought home for children. *The Modern Law Review* 1999; **62**:350—70:370.
11 This is articulated in international instruments such as the United Nations Convention on the Rights of the Child (20. xi. 1989; TS 44; Cm 1976) and in national legislation such as the Children Act 1989 and its equivalents in other UK jurisdictions, see chapters 2 and 3.
12 United Nations Convention on the Rights of the Child (20. xi. 1989; TS 44; Cm 1976).
13 In particular: Children Act 1989; The Children (Northern Ireland) Order 1995; Children (Scotland) Act 1991.
14 British Paediatric Association. *A paediatrician's brief guide to the UN Convention on the Rights of the Child.* London: BPA, 1995.
15 The BMA has also published several reports focusing on the effects of poverty and deprivation on health. British Medical Association. *Growing up in Britain: ensuring a healthy future for our children. A study of 0—5 year olds.* London: BMJ Books, 1999. British Medical Association. *Inequalities in health.* London: BMA, 1995. British Medical Association. *Deprivation and ill-health. British Medical Association Board of Science and Education discussion paper.* London: BMA, 1987.
16 British Association for Community Child Health, Royal College of Nursing, the International Child Health Group and the Children's Rights Development Unit. *Child health rights: implementing the UN Convention on the Rights of the Child within the National Health Service. A practitioners' guide.* London: BACCH, 1995.
17 World Medical Association. Declaration of Ottawa on the Rights of the Child to Health Care. 50th World Medical Assembly, Ottawa, October 1998. World Medical Association statements represent a consensus opinion among national medical associations. They are intended to provide general guidance but are not binding in the same way as international instruments that governments have ratified.
18 Alderson P, Montgomery J. *Health care choices: making decisions with children.* London: Institute for Public Policy Research, 1996.
19 Re M (Child: Refusal of Medical Treatment) [1999] 2 FLR 1097, [1999] 2 FCR 577.
20 Re M (Child: Refusal of Medical Treatment) [1999] 2 FLR 1097 at 1100C-D.
21 Re M (Child: Refusal of Medical Treatment) [1999] 2 FLR 1097 at 1100G.
22 Re W (A Minor) (Medical Treatment: Court's Jurisdiction) [1993] Fam 64, [1992] 3 WLR 758 at 776, [1992] 4 All ER 627, CA.
23 Re C (A Child) (HIV Testing) [1999] 2 FLR 1004, [2000] Fam Law 16, CA. This and some other examples of cases in which parental choice has been limited are discussed more fully in chapter 2.
24 United Nations Convention on the Rights of the Child (20. xi. 1989; TS 44; Cm 1976): Article 6.
25 United Nations Convention on the Rights of the Child (20. xi. 1989; TS 44; Cm 1976): Article 24.
26 See British Medical Association, Law Society. *Assessment of mental capacity: guidance for doctors and lawyers.* London: BMA, 1995.
27 Alderson P, Montgomery J. *Health care choices: making decisions with children.* London: Institute for Public Policy Research, 1996: 8—9.
28 Nelson LJ, Rushton CH, Cranford RE, Nelson RM, Glover JJ, Truog RD. Forgoing medically provided nutrition and hydration in paediatric patients. *Journal of Law, Medicine and Ethics* 1995;**23**:33—46:38.
29 Dunn J. *The beginnings of social understanding.* Oxford: Blackwell, 1988.
30 Rutter M. *Changing youth in a changing society: patterns of adolescent development*

and disorder. London: Nuffield Provincial Hospitals Trust and Cambridge, Mass: Harvard University Press, 1980; Rutter M. *Developing minds: challenge and continuity across the lifespan.* Harmondsworth: Penguin and New York: Basic Books, 1993.

2: The law on children, consent and medical treatment: England, Wales and Northern Ireland

The reasons for obtaining consent before providing medical treatment are ethical, clinical and legal. Seeking consent ensures that patients are involved in decisions about their care. Agreement and cooperation are often essential to a successful clinical outcome, and in law valid consent legitimises what otherwise would be unlawful conduct. The previous chapter looked at the ethical and good practice issues, and the purpose of this chapter is to describe the legal issues. It also gives some background about how the law has developed in England, Wales and Northern Ireland. Scottish law is discussed separately in chapter 3.

In England, Wales and Northern Ireland, much of the law affecting consent is not set out in legislation but is common (judge-made) law. In deciding cases, judges follow the precedents set in previous cases and the common law is the rules that are extracted from those decisions. Legal cases about the medical treatment of children usually involve a dispute and the situations are complex and difficult. They arise, for example, where the parties to the decision cannot reach agreement, or the proposed intervention is not for the therapeutic benefit of the child. They are not the situations faced in everyday practice, and although judges explain their reasoning, the courts' role is to resolve the particular situation rather than to provide guidance for future cases. General legal principles do emerge, but doctors must be guarded about applying these in circumstances that the courts have not considered, without first having taken legal advice.

The courts are almost always asked to settle a very specific matter, for example to authorise or reject a particular treatment.

This type of stark choice is unusual in medicine, where more often there are a number of people considering a range of options. Balancing the legal authority to rely on the consent of just one of the parties legally entitled to give it, with the moral imperative to discuss, consult and reach agreement, is the key issue in this book.

There is a further need for caution about the law in this area because all the court decisions described in this book were made before the rights and freedoms guaranteed under the European Convention on Human Rights[1] (the "Convention rights") were given effect in UK law by the Human Rights Act 1998. Since the Act took full effect on 2 October 2000, public authorities have been required to apply the Convention rights in all aspects of their activities. Previously the primary legal question was whether a proposed course of action was lawful. Now doctors and other public authorities must also assess whether their actions involve a person's human rights and, if so, whether they can legitimately be interfered with. The implications of this cannot, at the time of writing, be known. It may be that the decisions reached by health professionals in everyday practice and by the courts in extreme cases will be little affected, even though the basis of those decisions could be radically different. If there is any doubt about whether a course of action is compatible with the Convention rights, or whether there are clear and proper reasons for contravening any rights, doctors should seek legal advice. Information about relevant developments in this area will be put on the BMA's website.

2.1 When treatment can be given

Except in cases of emergency or incapacity, it is usually a patient's consent that allows medical treatment to be given. In the care of children, consent can come from any one of a number of sources; a competent young patient, parents (and in some circumstances other carers) or the courts. In England, Wales and Northern Ireland, the legal right of people to give consent for treatment on behalf of a young person is not wholly extinguished until the young person reaches 18.[2]

Where consent is unavailable and the situation is an emergency, it is lawful for doctors to give treatment to promote a child's best interests. An emergency is best described as a situation where the requirement for treatment is so pressing that there is not time to refer the matter to court.

It is also lawful as well as, in our view, ethically justifiable, to administer life-saving treatment against the wishes of a child or his or her parents if the situation is an emergency and any delay would lead to serious harm or even death. If time permits, however, there must be attempts at resolution before the family's wishes are overridden. Legal advice should be sought and usually the courts should be involved.[3]

2.2 Consent from competent young people

In England, Wales and Northern Ireland the age of majority is 18. Once a person reaches adulthood he or she has the exclusive right to give consent to treatment, and may also refuse proposed interventions. Adult patients are presumed competent to give consent until the contrary is shown. Currently, no one can give consent on behalf of an adult who is not competent to make treatment decisions, and doctors can lawfully treat adults unable to consent only if treatment is necessary and judged to be in that person's best interests.[4]

Although they do not acquire full adult rights to make their own decisions until they are 18, young people between 16 and 18 are also presumed to be competent to give consent, and should be treated as such unless there is evidence to suggest otherwise (although an expert government committee has recommended that the presumption should arise at age 10 or 12, see section 7.3). The law says that the

> consent of a minor who has attained the age of sixteen years to any surgical, medical or dental treatment which, in the absence of consent, would constitute a trespass to his person, shall be as effective as it would be if he were of full age; and where a minor has by virtue of this section given an effective consent to any treatment it shall not be necessary to obtain any consent for it from his parent or guardian.[5]

Surgical, medical or dental treatment in this context includes diagnosis and procedures ancillary to treatment, such as anaesthesia.[6] It is also assumed to extend to preventive measures intended to benefit health, such as immunisation.

No statute governs the rights of people under 16 to give consent to medical treatment. The issue was tested in the early 1980s, in a case where the courts were asked to rule on the rights of parents in respect of their children.[7]

The *Gillick* case

Mrs Gillick took her local health authority to court because it refused to assure her that her five daughters, all under 16, would not be given contraceptive advice and treatment without her knowledge and consent. The case followed the publication of a Department of Health and Social Security circular that advised that doctors consulted at a family planning clinic by a girl under 16 would not be acting unlawfully if they prescribed contraceptives, provided that they acted in good faith and to protect the young woman from the harmful effects of sexual intercourse. In seeking a declaration that this advice was unlawful, Mrs Gillick argued that a young girl's consent was legally ineffective and inconsistent with parental rights. She said that it was therefore necessary to involve parents.

This argument was rejected by the House of Lords where the majority opinion was that the relevant test was whether the girl had reached an age where she had "sufficient understanding and intelligence to enable her to understand fully what was proposed".[8] If she had, a doctor would not be acting unlawfully in giving advice and treatment.

Gillick v West Norfolk and Wisbech AHA

In reaching this decision, the judges also held that "parental rights were recognised by the law only as long as they were needed for the protection of the child and such rights yielded to the child's right to make his own decisions when he reached a sufficient understanding and intelligence to be capable of making up his own mind. Accordingly, a girl under 16 did not, merely by reason of her age, lack legal capacity to consent to contraceptive advice and treatment by a doctor".[9] Lord Fraser said it seemed to him to be "verging on the absurd to suggest that a boy or girl aged 15 could not effectively consent, for example, to have a medical examination of some trivial injury to his body or even to have a broken arm set".[10]

This judgment rejected the previously held notion that the

consent of parents is always needed before treating children and young people. Where a young person who has sufficient understanding and intelligence to understand fully what is proposed gives consent to treatment, consent from parents is not legally necessary although parental involvement should generally be encouraged. Nevertheless, treatment may proceed without their knowledge or against their wishes if the child cannot be persuaded to include them. It is widely accepted that the *Gillick* judgment also implied that a competent child is owed the same duty of confidentiality as any adult patient. This view is reflected in the guidance of professional and regulatory bodies, which do not distinguish between the rights of competent children and competent adults to confidentiality (see chapter 3).[11]

2.2.1 Limits on young people's rights to choose

At its time, the *Gillick* decision was regarded as a watershed: it appeared to clarify the issues around competent young people's consent to medical treatment by confirming their rights in law to act autonomously in decisions about their health care. In a 1990 publication, for example, renowned authors on children's rights commented that "[a]s a result of this decision it seems that, provided the 'maturity test' is satisfied, parents can neither compel nor prevent medical treatment".[12] A right to refuse treatment seemed to most a logical extension of a right to consent and the law appeared to be dealing with competent young people as it would with adults. In subsequent cases where young people have refused treatment, however, this has not been borne out.

Several important cases indicate the ambivalence society has about allowing young people to refuse treatment. (Some of these are discussed in more detail in other chapters.) The first reported time the rights of a mature minor to refuse treatment were discussed in court was in 1991.[13]

Refusal of treatment: the case of R

R was a 15-year-old girl who refused anti-psychotic treatment. She had poor and sometimes violent relationships with her parents and appeared to experience visual and auditory hallucinations and sometimes suicidal thoughts. But she also experienced periods of lucidity, brought about by drug therapy. During these intervals her doctors believed that she had the necessary competence to make decisions about her treatment. The local authority initiated wardship proceedings to obtain the authority to provide anti-psychotic treatment whether or not R consented.

The Court of Appeal held that R was not competent to give consent, and authorised the treatment against her wishes.

Re R (A Minor) (Wardship: Consent to Treatment)

Although in the court's view R lacked competence, Lord Donaldson said that a "*Gillick* competent" child

can consent, but if he or she declines to do so or refuses, consent can be given by someone else who has parental rights or responsibilities. The failure or refusal of the "Gillick competent" child is a very important factor in the doctor's decision whether or not to treat, but does not prevent the necessary consent being obtained from another competent source.[14]

In other words, the Court of Appeal was of the opinion that the rights of parents and others to give consent are not extinguished when a young person is competent to give consent for him or herself. A year later, another case came to court where the patient was presumed to have the competence to give consent because she was 16.[15] The question arose about whether a young person's statutory right to give consent was exclusive or shared with parents or the court. In both these cases, the court referred to the provision of the Family Law Reform Act 1969, which, in the same section as making clear that a person of 16's consent is as valid as that of an adult, goes on to state that "[n]othing in this section shall be construed as making ineffective any consent which would have been effective if this section had not been enacted".[16]

Refusal of treatment: the case of W

W was 16 years old and living in a specialist adolescent residential unit under local authority care. Her physical condition due to anorexia nervosa deteriorated to the extent that the authority wished to transfer her to a specialist hospital for treatment. W refused, wanting instead to stay where she was and to cure herself when she decided it was right to do so. The local authority applied to court to be allowed to move W and for authorisation that she could be given medical treatment without her consent if necessary.

The judge in the Family Division of the High Court concluded that W was competent to make a decision to refuse treatment and that the court could, in exercising its inherent jurisdiction, override a refusal of medical treatment by a competent young person if that was in her best interests.

W appealed against the decision. Her condition significantly deteriorated, and the Court of Appeal made an emergency order enabling her to be taken to and treated at a specialist hospital notwithstanding her lack of consent. In delivering its judgment, the Court of Appeal held that the Family Division judge had been wrong to conclude that W was competent, since a desire not to be treated was symptomatic of anorexia nervosa. The court also said that its inherent powers were theoretically limitless and that there was no doubt that it had power to override the refusal of a minor, whether over the age of 16 or under that age but "*Gillick* competent".[17]

Re W (A Minor)
(Medical Treatment: Court's Jurisdiction)

In this case Lord Donaldson described consent as a legal "flak jacket"

which protects the doctor from claims by the litigious whether he acquires it from his patient, who may be a minor over the age of 16 or a "Gillick competent" child under that age, or from another person having parental responsibilities which include a right to consent to treatment of the minor. Anyone who gives him a flak jacket (ie consent) may take it back, but the doctor only needs one and so long as he continues to have one he has the legal right to proceed.[18]

In neither of these cases were the young people found by the court to be competent and so the views of the judges that the court or a parent could override a competent refusal are not necessarily binding on future decisions. They are, however, likely to be strongly influential in cases of young people refusing essential treatment.

Despite allowing a young person's refusal to be overridden, the courts have been clear that a young person's wishes are important in the determination of his or her best interests. In *Re W*, for example, the Court of Appeal stressed that competent young people should generally not be subjected to invasive treatment against their wishes without the authorisation of a court.[19]

In a subsequent, and controversial, High Court case it was suggested that there is no need to obtain consent from a court where consent from a parent is forthcoming.[20] In *Re K, W and H*, a hospital was criticised for seeking an order to authorise the provision of "emergency" medication to a number of 15-year-old children who were subject to secure accommodation orders.

Parental consent: the case of K, W and H

Three young people, K, W and H were the subjects of secure accommodation orders in a hospital's secure adolescent unit. The parents of all three had given their consent to treatment. The hospital authority applied to the High Court for orders under the Children Act to authorise the provision of "emergency" medication to these patients in keeping with its policy of doing so where there was doubt about a young person's ability to consent.

Referring back to the judgment in *Re R*, the application was refused as being "misconceived and unnecessary" since the hospital was lawfully entitled to proceed with treatment based on the authority of parental consent. This was held to be the case even if the young people themselves refused the treatment.

Re K, W and H (Minors) (Medical Treatment)

This decision seems contrary to the recommendation in *Re W* that the courts' view should be sought before imposing treatment upon a child who may be competent. It leaves uncertainty about the extent to which it is necessary to seek court approval before proceeding. In such cases, doctors should approach their lawyers for advice about their authority to proceed and whether there is a benefit in bringing a case before the court (see section 2.5).

2.2.2 A statutory right to refuse

Children have a statutory right to refuse to submit to medical or psychiatric examination or other assessment that has been directed by the courts for the purpose of an interim care, supervision, child protection or emergency protection order, provided that the child "is of sufficient understanding to make an informed decision".[21] Whether the courts' inherent jurisdiction could override this statutory right to refuse was tested in the case of *South Glamorgan County Council v W and B* (also discussed in section 7.4.2).[22]

A statutory right to refuse: the case of A

A was 15 and had longstanding behavioural problems. She confined herself to the front room of her father's house with the curtains drawn for approximately 11 months, and was described as indulging in obsessive behaviour and being demanding and domineering towards her father and aunt who cared for her. The local authority commenced care proceedings, and a care order was made with a direction for her to receive psychiatric examination and assessment under the Children Act. She refused to give consent to this, and the local authority brought proceedings to ask the High Court to exercise its inherent jurisdiction to override A's refusal.

Despite finding her competent, the judge ruled that there was power under the inherent jurisdiction to override the refusal of a person under 18 years of age to submit to psychiatric assessment and examination, even where the Children Act made specific provision that the refusal of a competent young person should be respected.

South Glamorgan County Council v W and B

The court held that its "jurisdiction over minors was unlimited and had not been abrogated by the Children Act 1989".[23] The decision has been criticised, with legal experts such as Kennedy and Grubb, for example, commenting that "it is not easy to reconcile this view of the law with the principle that prerogative power yields to inconsistent statutory provisions".[24] Doctors asked to examine a competent young person for the purpose of a care, supervision or emergency protection order should seek legal advice if he or she refuses.

2.2.3 Comment on the law

The state of the law is the subject of much academic debate, and its apparent inconsistencies can be confusing for practitioners, patients and carers. To some commentators the power to refuse is the partner of the power to give consent, and it is logically inconsistent to credit competent children with only one half of this pair. Kennedy has said that cases since *Gillick* have "driven a coach and horses" through that House of Lords decision.[25] It has been argued that judges should not go through the pretence of saying that young people can make those decisions they are competent to make, but that instead the law "should openly declare that welfare reigns when grave decisions with momentous outcomes are considered and recognise that adolescent autonomy is, inevitably, circumscribed".[26]

Another criticism of the "retreat from *Gillick*" is the formidably high degree of proof of competence the law demands of young people who refuse treatment. Although people under 18 can and do regularly give consent to complex and risky procedures, the law generally finds that young people refusing treatment do not meet the courts' standards for competence to refuse. Some distinction between consent and refusal is, however, defensible. When giving consent to proposed treatment, the patient is accepting the advice of a qualified professional. Refusal, on the other hand, is a rejection of expert advice from a necessarily less well-informed position and may have grave consequences, both in terms of the immediate physical effects of non-treatment and the possible closing down of options for future treatment. Other commentators have therefore commended the courts' position on refusal as simply interpreting the Family Law Reform Act, which preserves the right of others to consent.[27]

The BMA's view is that there is a need for clarity about when it is acceptable to override a young person's wishes and when it is not. The legal issues could be clarified by the courts or statute, and would be an appropriate subject for consideration by the Law Commission particularly in the light of the Human Rights Act which may have implications for young people's refusals of treatment. Meanwhile, this book is the Association's attempt to provide as much guidance as it is presently possible to do. Additional guidance, as it becomes available, will be posted on the BMA's website.

2.3 Consent from parents and people with parental responsibility

2.3.1 Parental responsibility

Parental responsibility consists of the rights, duties, powers, responsibilities and authority that parents have, by law, in respect of their child and his or her property, and includes the right to give consent to medical treatment.[28] The right to a family life in the European Convention on Human Rights entitles parents to be involved in decisions relating to their children,[29] and it is arguable that depriving parents of involvement breaches their rights to be free from inhuman or degrading treatment.[30] The rules about parental responsibility are described below, but if there is any doubt about whether the person giving consent is lawfully entitled to do so, and in particular if the family does not have its permanent home in England, Wales or Northern Ireland so that different rules may apply, doctors should seek further advice from professional and indemnifying bodies and their lawyers if necessary.

A child's biological parents are the child's legal parents, unless the child has been adopted or was born as the result of some methods of assisted reproduction. Where the child has been adopted, the adopters are the child's legal parents. Where the child has been born as a result of assisted reproduction, there are rules under the Human Fertilisation and Embryology Act 1990 that determine the child's legal parentage.

Not all parents, however, have parental responsibility. Both parents have parental responsibility if they were married at the time of the child's conception, or birth, or at some time after the child's birth. Neither parent loses parental responsibility if they divorce.

If the parents have never married, only the mother automatically has parental responsibility. The father may acquire it by entering into a parental responsibility agreement with the mother and registering it in the Principal Registry of the Family Division of the High Court, or through a parental responsibility order made by a court.

The Government has announced its intention to amend these rules, following a consultation exercise carried out in 1998 by the Lord Chancellor's Department, so that parental responsibility is automatically conferred on unmarried fathers who sign the child's birth certificate along with the mother. This requires a change in legislation and, at the time of writing, it has not been established when these changes will take place. The BMA will put information about any changes to the rules on its website. The Human Rights Act may also affect the range of people entitled to be involved in, and make decisions for, children. In interpreting the European Convention on Human Rights, the European Court of Human Rights has accepted a broad definition of "family life" that does not distinguish between families according to their status, including whether or not the partners are married.[31] There is also an argument that depriving unmarried fathers of parental responsibility contravenes the Convention right to freedom from discrimination, although commentators have said this is unlikely.[32]

A person other than a child's biological parents can acquire parental responsibility by being appointed as the child's guardian (an appointment usually takes effect on the death of the parents) or by having a residence order made in his or her favour, when parental responsibility lasts for the duration of the order. A local authority acquires parental responsibility (shared with the parents) while the child is the subject of a care order.

2.3.2 Limits on parental rights

It is not always clear whether the likely medical benefits of treatment outweigh its burdens, and in such cases, parents are well placed and equipped to weigh the medical advice and apply it to their child's circumstances. The courts have emphasised that usually parents make the right decision about their child's best interests, and most decision making is, rightly, left to children and parents with appropriate input from the clinical team.[33] Accordingly, a court invited to override the wishes of parents will be extremely cautious, and will only do so where it is clearly in the child's best interests. For example, such a decision might be made if parents refuse an intervention that would provide a clear benefit to the child or if the statistical chances of recovery are good. In the case described below, the High Court overrode a mother's refusal to allow her baby to be tested for HIV (this case is also discussed in 1.4.5 and 3.3.2.).[34]

Whether to test C for HIV

C was five months old when a case was brought by her local authority for a specific issue order to allow her to be given a blood test to determine her HIV status. The child's

---

mother had known she was infected with HIV at the time of C's delivery by natural water-birth. The mother had refused to accept advice about medication towards the end of pregnancy and the benefits of Caesarean delivery, and continued to breast-feed her baby, despite medical advice about the risks of transmission of infection. Her GP recommended HIV testing to establish whether C was infected, and based on that information, to plan for C's management and care.

The parents, who favoured complementary therapies and objected to any conventional therapy, contended that it had not been established that HIV was truly a virus, nor that it was the sole cause of AIDS. They also dismissed the possibility of transmission of the infection to C by breast-feeding.

The court held that testing would clearly be in C's best interests, that overall the advantage of the proposed test was very substantial and the case for testing overwhelming. Permission to appeal was refused.

Re C (A Child) (HIV Testing)

In this case, the medical evidence was unambiguous. Knowing C's HIV status would help her doctors to protect her from the risk of infection and to provide appropriate care and treatment. A similar dilemma was faced by the courts in a case where a young person, able to be involved in treatment decisions together with his parents, refused a life-saving blood transfusion.[35]

Refusal of blood transfusion: the case of A

A was nearly 16 years old, and suffering from leukaemia. He urgently needed a blood transfusion as a life-saving measure. He and his parents, however, had refused consent to this, being devout Jehovah's Witnesses. Although the boy knew that he would die if he did not receive the transfusion, nobody had told him how prolonged and painful his death would be. The judge in the High Court therefore concluded that whilst he clearly had sufficient intelligence to be capable of making decisions about his own wellbeing, there was still a range of decisions the full implications of which A was still insufficiently mature to grasp.[36] Thus, it was concluded, he lacked the competence to refuse.

The judge described how he put himself in the position of the "ordinary father and mother" to reach a decision, based on A's welfare that included A's own wishes (as required by the Children Act) together with the particular circumstances and the religious community within which he lived. In this context, it was ruled that leave should be given to the hospital to carry out such treatment as was deemed appropriate, including blood transfusions.

Following the case, A continued to express his rejection of treatment, and when he reached adulthood, he exercised his right to refuse further transfusions and died.

Re E (A Minor) (Wardship: Medical Treatment)

Again in this case, the evidence was clear that the refused procedure had a good chance of clinical success. If, on the other hand, treatment is contrary to the child's clinical interests the courts are unlikely to uphold a request for it to be continued. In the case of *Re C* below, the High Court was asked to intervene where parents asked for treatment that the health team believed was inappropriate.[37]

Withdrawal of treatment: the case of C

C was a 16-month-old girl, suffering from spinal muscular atrophy, a progressive disease that causes severe emaciation and disability. She was dependent on intermittent positive pressure ventilation. Her doctors sought authority from the High Court to withdraw the ventilation, and to not reinstate it or resuscitate C if she suffered further respiratory relapse. They maintained that further treatment would cause her increasing distress, could cause medical complications, and could do little more than delay death without significant alleviation of suffering.

The judge described C's parents as highly responsible orthodox Jews, who loved their daughter but who were unable to "bring themselves to face the inevitable future".[38] The doctor's treatment plan of withholding resuscitation and ventilation and providing palliative care was endorsed by the judge to "ease her suffering and permit her life to end peacefully".[39]

Re C (A Minor) (Medical Treatment)

Despite the courts' usual acceptance of the medical advice where this shows a clear route to follow, there has been one reported case where the courts upheld parental refusal against the health team's recommendation.[40]

Parental refusal: the case of C

C suffered from biliary atresia, a liver defect, and was not expected to live beyond two and a half years without a liver transplant. He had undergone major invasive surgery when he was three and a half weeks old that was unsuccessful and appeared to cause him severe pain and distress. Both of C's parents were health professionals experienced in caring for young sick children.

C's mother argued that she did not want to expose her son to further distress and believed that it would be best for him to be cared for by her abroad, where his father was working. C was referred to a hospital carrying out liver transplants, but when an organ became available, C and his mother were abroad and could not be contacted. When they returned to England, the mother continued to oppose the operation.

The local authority asked the court to exercise its inherent jurisdiction to order that a transplant would be in C's best interests, to give permission to perform the surgery and to order that C be returned to England for the surgery. The Court of Appeal disagreed, and held that it would not be in C's best interests to give consent and require him to be returned to the jurisdiction for the operation.

C later had the transplant with his mother's consent.

Re T (A Minor) (Wardship: Medical Treatment)

In deciding the case, Lord Justice Waite stated that

the greater the scope for genuine debate between one view and another [about the best interests of the child] the stronger will be the inclination of the court to be influenced by a reflection that in the last analysis the best interests of every child include an expectation that difficult decisions affecting the length and quality of its life will be taken for it by the parent to whom its care has been entrusted by nature.[41]

The clinical evidence was unchallenged: C was very likely to die before he was three years old without a transplant and his doctors were optimistic that a transplant would give C many years of life and normal growth and development. C's welfare had to be the determining factor in the court's decision, but the judges recognised that his welfare depended on his mother who would be expected to care for him, probably alone since the father was abroad, through surgery and for many years afterwards. The court was apparently influenced by the parents being health professionals and the practical difficulties of ensuring compliance, particularly since the family was abroad. The decision may have been very different in different social circumstances, and the court's decision is controversial. It is perhaps clear that the courts would not follow this precedent in cases that do not follow such particular circumstances. Doctors should seek legal advice if they are concerned about the willingness of parents to provide essential care following invasive procedures.

2.4 Consent from carers

Apart from people with parental responsibility, any person who has care of a child, for example a grandparent or child minder, may do "what is reasonable in all the circumstances of the case for the purpose of safeguarding or promoting the child's welfare".[42] This could include giving consent to medical treatment. Parents are also entitled to authorise another person to take over particular responsibilities.[43] This might be because parents have arranged for somebody else to look after their child while they are away. It is unlikely to be reasonable for a non-parent to give consent if he or she knows that the child's parents are likely to object, and treatment should only be given in such circumstances if the situation is an emergency and delay would lead to serious harm or death. If a carer brings a child for treatment, steps should be taken to ascertain the parents' views, and if there is doubt about authority to proceed, doctors should seek legal advice.

2.5 Consent from the courts

The courts have the power to give consent to treatment on behalf of a person under 18. Court involvement is necessary in only a minority of cases, since most decisions are of the type doctors and families are entitled to make and usually agreement is reached by the child, the people with parental responsibility and the health care team. Their goal is the same — to benefit the child — and in the vast majority of cases it is possible to agree on the best route to achieve this. If, however, agreement cannot be reached in a reasonable time period, which will depend on the nature and likely course of the patient's condition, lawyers might advise that it is necessary to seek legal review. The courts have also indicated that interventions of certain types, for example decisions about sterilisation, organ donation and circumcision where the parents disagree, should be referred to court. Section 2.5.3 discusses situations in which the courts should have an input.

Going to court can be distressing for those concerned and it is essential that ongoing support is provided for the child, parents, other relatives and carers and the health care team. In general, less confrontational means of problem solving are preferable. There are great benefits, however, of a legal system that can give rulings very quickly where necessary. This is an important safeguard for young people and their carers.

2.5.1 Mechanisms for court involvement

There are two mechanisms (known as "jurisdictions") that can be invoked to resolve disputes about medical treatment for children: the Children Act and the inherent jurisdiction of the High Court with respect to children. These are described briefly below, and entitle the court to override the wishes of any other person in relation to the child, including the child him or herself. Proceedings under either mechanism may be instituted by an interested party, which could be a health professional involved in the child's care or, more likely, an NHS trust, health authority or local authority. Doctors should approach their lawyers for advice on this matter.

Under the Children Act and Children (Northern Ireland) Order, the courts can invoke statutory provisions to authorise or prohibit steps taken in the exercise of parental responsibility in relation to medical treatment. They do this through their powers to make specific issue and prohibited steps orders. A specific issue order is "an order giving directions for the purpose of determining a specific question which has arisen, or which may arise, in connection with any aspect of parental responsibility for a child".[44] Its purpose is to resolve a situation in which there is disagreement over the exercise of parental responsibility. A prohibited steps order, on the other hand, is "an order that no step which could be taken by a parent in meeting his parental responsibility for a child, and which is of a kind specified in the order, shall be taken by any person without the consent of the court".[45] This prevents the exercise of parental responsibility in a particular way without the consent of the courts. The courts may not intervene by making an order unless to do so is better for the child than there being no order.[46]

In addition to powers under the Children Act and Children (Northern Ireland) Order, the High Court has ancient, non-statutory (inherent) jurisdiction over children. This jurisdiction is "theoretically unlimited"[47] and means the courts can authorise medical treatment (give valid consent) or forbid a course of action if this is in the child's best interests.

The inherent jurisdiction is broad, and embraces things that parents do not have the power to do. The High Court can make orders that require third parties to act in a particular way. For example, a doctor might be authorised to carry out or forbidden from carrying out proposed treatment, although no court will order a doctor to provide treatment that is contrary to his or her clinical judgment (see section 2.5.3). The High Court can also prevent the media from revealing the identity of, or information about, any medical treatment a child may be undergoing or may undergo in the future.

Another arm of the inherent jurisdiction means that a child may be made a ward of the High Court. Wardship is best thought of as a special status conferred upon a child by the inherent jurisdiction, a status that places the custody of the child in the court so that no important step in the child's life may be taken without the leave of the court. Wardship proceedings are started, like proceedings under the inherent jurisdiction, by issuing an originating summons. Once the summons has been issued, the child is immediately in the care of the court and no important steps may be taken without the court's permission. This endures for 21 days, after which time it will lapse unless an application is made to the court for a decision on its continuation.

In matters of great urgency, the High Court is available at all hours. Outside normal office hours, contact should be made, normally by a lawyer, with the security officer at the Royal Courts of Justice. He or she contacts the designated urgent business officer by telephone, whose responsibility it is to assess the urgency of the application and, if appropriate, to contact the duty judge. The judge may deal with the matter over the telephone, or may direct attendance at his or her home or lodgings on circuit. Lawyers may therefore find it prudent to have a medical expert available to speak to the judge in such circumstances. The judge may appoint a guardian *ad litem* to act for, and safeguard the interests of, the child.

2.5.2 Welfare and proportionality

When a court determines any matter relating to the upbringing of a child, it is required by law to have the child's welfare as the paramount consideration.[48] A checklist of factors relevant to a child's welfare is given in statute and includes:

(a) *the ascertainable wishes and feelings of the child concerned (considered in the light of his age and understanding);*

(b) *his physical, emotional and educational needs;*

(c) *the likely effect on him of any change in his circumstances;*

(d) *his age, sex, background and any characteristics of his which the court considers relevant;*

(e) *any harm which he has suffered or is at risk of suffering; and*

(f) *how capable each of his parents, and any other person in relation to whom the court considers the question to be relevant, is of meeting his needs.*[49]

The courts are also required to apply the rights and freedoms of the European Convention on Human Rights, which include freedom from inhuman or degrading treatment, rights to life, a fair trial, privacy, family life, and freedom of religion.[50] The Convention rights apply to children as they do to adults, and the European courts have accepted the importance of children's wishes and feelings in determining applications about them. The aim is a fair balance between the protection of individuals' fundamental rights and the demands of society, and any interference with the rights of a person or group must be proportionate with the intended objective. The courts must interpret statute in a way that, as far as possible, is compatible with these Convention rights and are also entitled to overturn a decided matter of common law that would otherwise be binding under the ordinary rules of precedent, where this is necessary to comply with the Convention.[51]

2.5.3 When to go to court

Doctors should approach their lawyers for advice if there is doubt about whether a course of action is lawful. Whilst it is neither helpful nor desirable to draw up a definitive list of situations that should be taken to court, some generalisations can be made to help doctors to identify when they should seek legal advice.

Legal advice should be sought when:

- agreement over how to proceed cannot be reached (for example where consent is refused by the holders of parental responsibility);
- a competent young person refuses invasive treatment;
- administering treatment against the wishes of a competent young person would require the use of restraint or force;
- it is not clear whether the people with parental responsibility are acting in the best interests of the child;
- the proposed care is beyond the scope of parental consent because it is controversial or non-therapeutic (for example sterilisation, organ donation and circumcision if parents disagree);
- the courts require legal review of the decision;
- the treatment requires detention outwith the provisions of mental health legislation;
- the people with parental responsibility lack the competence to make the decision;
- the child is a ward of court and the proposed step is important; or
- the proposed course of action might breach a person's Convention rights.

The role of the court is to determine where the child's best interests lie and this may result in authorising doctors to treat. The courts do not have the power to require a doctor to treat.

> *No doctor can be required to treat a child, whether by the court in the exercise of its wardship jurisdiction, by the parents, by the child or anyone else. The decision whether to treat is dependent upon an exercise of his own professional judgment, subject only to the threshold requirement that, save in exceptional cases usually of emergency, he has the consent of someone who has the authority to give that consent.*[52]

Thus, whilst the authorisation of a court tells doctors that treatment is lawful, it does not mean that treatment must definitely go ahead. The courts can give "leave" to carry out a particular procedure or treatment, and doctors must then assess whether treatment is appropriate and whether it is in the child's best interests (see chapter 1).

2.6 Summary

Decisions about whether to accept or reject medical treatment should ideally be taken by children together with their parents, although competent young people do have the option of seeking and obtaining medical treatment independently.

Consent for the treatment of a person under 18 can come from any one of the following:

- a competent child;
- a person or local authority with parental responsibility;
- a court; or
- a person caring for a child but only if it is reasonable in the circumstances to safeguard or promote the child's welfare.

With consent from any one of the above, health professionals are protected from a charge of battery, even if one of the others refuses the treatment (although consent, of course, does not exclude liability for negligence). Consent does not necessarily mean that treatment must be given. Doctors have legal and ethical obligations over and above the requirement to obtain valid consent, and should not proceed if, in their clinical judgment, giving treatment is inappropriate. At the core of these obligations is respect for human rights.

Whoever gives consent for the treatment, the child's wishes are an essential part of assessing what is in his or her best interests. Competent, sustained wishes should not be overridden lightly, and all children should be offered the opportunity for their views to be heard and given due consideration.

The rights of children and their parents to refuse treatment is limited. Parents are not entitled to refuse treatment that, in the view of the court, it is in the child's best interests to have. Similarly, a competent young person's refusal might be overridden in certain circumstances. The BMA accepts that the level of competence necessary to refuse treatment that may prolong or significantly enhance life is very high and that in some cases even a competent refusal may not be determinative where its consequences are extremely grave. A refusal by a competent young person may, however, tip the balance in favour of withholding treatment in certain circumstances, notwithstanding consent from a parent or court. Refusal of treatment is discussed further in chapter 6.

Without consent, or even against the wishes of the child or parents, emergency treatment may be provided if any delay would lead to death or serious harm. Doctors should consult their lawyers as soon as practicable.

References

1 Convention for the Protection of Human Rights and Fundamental Freedoms (4. ix. 1950; TS 71; Cmnd 8969).
2 Re W (A Minor) (Medical Treatment: Court's Jurisdiction) [1993] Fam 64, [1992] 3 WLR 758, [1992] 4 All ER 627, CA.
3 For example, two cases involving Jehovah's Witness children have suggested that the approval of a court should be sought before the administration of treatment where parents and children refuse. Re O (A Minor) (Medical Treatment) [1993] 2 FLR 149, [1993] 1 FCR 925, [1993] 4 Med LR 272; Re S (A Minor) (Medical Treatment) [1993] 1 FLR 377, [1993] Fam Law 215.
4 Since the early 1980s, the UK government has been considering reform of the law to allow the appointment of health care proxies who would be lawfully entitled to take decisions about health care. At the time of writing, these proposals continued to be under discussion. Information about developments in this area can be obtained from the BMA's medical ethics department and on the BMA web page (www.bma.org.uk).
5 Family Law Reform Act 1969 s8(1); Age of Majority Act (NI) 1969 art 4(1).
6 Family Law Reform Act 1969 s8(2); Age of Majority Act (NI) 1969 art 4(2).
7 Gillick v West Norfolk and Wisbech AHA [1986] AC 112, [1985] 3 WLR 830, [1985] 3 All ER 402, HL.
8 Gillick v West Norfolk and Wisbech AHA [1986] AC 112 at 114.
9 Gillick v West Norfolk and Wisbech AHA [1986] AC 112 at 113.
10 Gillick v West Norfolk and Wisbech AHA [1986] AC 112 at 169.
11 General Medical Council. Confidentiality: protecting and providing information. London: GMC, 2000.
12 Eekelaar J, Dingwell R. The reform of child care law: a practical guide to the Children Act 1989. London: Routledge, 1990: 24.
13 Re R (A Minor) (Wardship: Consent to Treatment) [1992] Fam 11, [1991] 3 WLR 592, [1992] 1 FLR 190, CA.
14 Re R (A Minor) (Wardship: Consent to Treatment) [1992] Fam 11 at 12.
15 Re W (A Minor) (Medical Treatment: Court's Jurisdiction) [1993] Fam 64, [1992] 3 WLR 758, [1992] 4 All ER 627, CA.
16 Family Law Reform Act 1969 s8(3); Age of Majority Act (NI) 1969 s4(3).
17 Re W (A Minor) (Medical Treatment: Court's Jurisdiction) [1993] Fam 64 at 81.
18 Re W (A Minor) (Medical Treatment: Court's Jurisdiction) [1993] Fam 64 at 78.
19 Re W (A Minor) (Medical Treatment: Court's Jurisdiction) [1993] Fam 64, [1992] 3 WLR 758, [1992] 4 All ER 627, CA.
20 Re K, W and H (Minors) (Medical Treatment) [1993] 1 FLR 854, 15 BMLR 60, [1993] Fam Law 280, [1993] 1 FCR 240.
21 Children Act 1989 s38(6); The Children (Northern Ireland) Order 1995 art 57(6).

22 South Glamorgan CC v B, sub nom South Glamorgan CC v W and B [1993] FLR 574, [1993] 1 FCR 626, [1993] Fam Law 398.

23 South Glamorgan CC v B, sub nom South Glamorgan CC v W and B [1993] FLR 574 at 583.

24 Kennedy I, Grubb A, eds. *Principles of medical law*. Oxford: Oxford University Press, 1998: 209.

25 Kennedy I. Consent to treatment: the capable person. In: Dyer C, ed. *Doctors, patients and the law*. Oxford: Blackwell Scientific Publications, 1992: 60.

26 Bridge C. Religious beliefs and teenage refusal of medical treatment. *The Modern Law Review* 1999;62:585—94:594.

27 Mason JK, McCall Smith RA. *Law and medical ethics*. London: Butterworths, 1999: 257—61.

28 Children Act 1989 s3(1); The Children (Northern Ireland) Order 1995 art 6(1).

29 W v United Kingdom Series A, No 121, (1987) 10 EHRR 29.

30 Kurt v Turkey (1998) EHRR 373 at para 134. For discussion, see also Fennell P. Withdrawal of life sustaining treatment for child without parental consent. *Medical Law Review* 2000;8:125—9.

31 Horowitz M, Kingscote G, Nicholls M. *The Human Rights Act 1998. A special bulletin for family lawyers*. London: Butterworths, 1999: 29.

32 Horowitz M, Kingscote G, Nicholls M. *The Human Rights Act 1998. A special bulletin for family lawyers*. London: Butterworths, 1999: 47.

33 Re T (A Minor) (Wardship: Medical Treatment) [1997] 1 WLR 242, [1997] 1 All ER 906, [1997] 1 FLR 502, CA.

34 Re C (A Child) (HIV Testing) [1999] 2 FLR 1004, [2000] Fam Law 16, CA.

35 Re E (A Minor) (Wardship: Medical Treatment) [1993] 1 FLR 386, [1994] 5 Med LR 73.

36 Re E (A Minor) (Wardship: Medical Treatment) [1993] 1 FLR 386.

37 Re C (A Minor) (Medical Treatment), sub nom Re C (A Minor) (Withdrawal of Lifesaving Treatment) [1998] 1 FLR 384, [1998] 1 FCR 1.

38 Re C (A Minor) (Medical Treatment), sub nom Re C (A Minor) (Withdrawal of Lifesaving Treatment) [1998] 1 FLR 384 at 386.

39 Re C (A Minor) (Medical Treatment), sub nom Re C (A Minor) (Withdrawal of Lifesaving Treatment) [1998] 1 FLR 384 at 391.

40 Re T (A Minor) (Wardship: Medical Treatment) [1997] 1 WLR 242, [1997] 1 All ER 906, [1997] 1 FLR 502, CA.

41 Re T (A Minor) (Wardship: Medical Treatment) [1997] 1 FLR 502 at 514, CA.

42 Children Act 1989 s3(5); The Children (Northern Ireland) Order 1995 art 6(5).

43 Children Act 1989 s2(9); The Children (Northern Ireland) Order 1995 art 5(8).

44 Children Act 1989 s8(1); The Children (Northern Ireland) Order 1995 art 8(1).

45 Children Act 1989 s8(1); The Children (Northern Ireland) Order 1995 art 8(1).

46 Children Act 1989 s1(5); The Children (Northern Ireland) Order 1995 art 3(5).

47 South Glamorgan CC v B, sub nom South Glamorgan CC v W and B [1993] FLR 574 at 584, [1993] 1 FCR 626, [1993] Fam Law 398.

48 Children Act 1989 s1(1); The Children (Northern Ireland) Order 1995 art 3(1).

49 Children Act 1989 s1(3); The Children (Northern Ireland) Order 1995 art 3(3).

50 Convention for the Protection of Human Rights and Fundamental Freedoms (4. ix. 1950; TS 71; Cmnd 8969): Articles 3, 2, 6, 8 and 9.

51 Horowitz M, Kingscote G, Nicholls M. *The Human Rights Act 1998. A special bulletin for family lawyers*. London: Butterworths, 1999: 8.

52 Re R (A Minor) (Wardship: Consent to Treatment) [1992] Fam 11 at 26.

3: The law on children, consent and medical treatment: Scotland

In contrast to the predominantly common law approach in England, Wales and Northern Ireland, in Scotland there is a greater emphasis on statutory provision for consent to medical treatment by young people. The Age of Legal Capacity (Scotland) Act 1991 sets out the age at which a person may give legally valid consent to various matters including medical treatment.[1] Other statutes, chiefly the Children (Scotland) Act 1995, cover situations in which the child or young person does not have the competence to give legally valid consent, or where there is a dispute between people with parental responsibility. The Children (Scotland) Act contains legal procedures to protect children and young people. The Adults with Incapacity (Scotland) Act 2000 concerns the treatment and welfare of people over 16 who are unable to give consent.[2]

Several of the statutory provisions have yet to be interpreted by the Scottish courts in the context of medical treatment, which leads to some uncertainty.[3] Guidance in interpretation may, however, be taken from the views of the Scottish Law Commission, which conducted wide ranging consultation before drafting the Bill that was subsequently enacted almost unaltered as the Age of Legal Capacity (Scotland) Act.[4] Where issues have not been considered by the Scottish courts, it is possible that cases heard in other UK jurisdictions, predominantly England, may be of assistance. Some such cases are mentioned here. Scottish civil courts, however, are not bound by English decisions where they are in conflict with principles of Scots law. English cases then have only persuasive authority at most. The House of Lords is the highest domestic court of appeal for most Scottish civil cases, but it must decide cases in accordance with the

Scottish law. Reference to cases decided outside Scotland are therefore made with caution, particularly where there appears to be divergence on important issues of principle, such as whether a competent young person can refuse medical treatment.

The law is also influenced by the European Convention on Human Rights[5] and case law from the European Court may influence the decisions of the Scottish courts. In devolving powers to the Scottish Parliament, the Scotland Act 1998 made specific reference to the need to comply with the Convention, so that an Act of the Scottish Parliament cannot include provisions that are incompatible with Convention rights as defined in the Human Rights Act 1998.[6] Furthermore, a member of the Scottish Executive has no power to make subordinate legislation or, indeed to do anything else, which would be incompatible with Convention rights.[7]

Therefore even before the implementation of the Human Rights Act, Acts of the Scottish Parliament were subject to scrutiny in respect of their potential impact on Convention rights. There are a number of ways in which challenges can be made in pre-enactment, and other scrutiny, procedures. It is expected that these will prevent the need for subsequent challenge, although a court or tribunal may still strike down a provision of an Act of the Scottish Parliament if it is considered to be in conflict with Convention rights. The provision would then be regarded as being outside the legislative competence of the Scottish Parliament and hence of no effect.

With the implementation of the Human Rights Act, British citizens will be able to enforce Convention rights directly in Scottish courts and they still have the right to apply to have their cases heard in the European Court of Human Rights in Strasbourg once domestic court proceedings have been exhausted.[8]

3.1 When treatment can be given

As in England, Wales and Northern Ireland, it is usually a patient's consent that allows medical treatment to be given. In the case of children, consent can come from any one of a number of sources: a competent young person, parents (and in some circumstances other carers) or the courts. In Scotland it appears that the legal rights of parents, carers and the courts to give consent may be extinguished when a young person is competent to decide for him or herself.[9]

Where consent is unavailable, for example in an emergency and the patient is unable to communicate, it is lawful for doctors to give treatment that is necessary to preserve life, health or wellbeing.[10] It is also lawful in Scotland to administer life-saving treatment against the wishes of a child or young person who is not competent to give consent, or against the wishes of any child's parents, if the situation is an emergency and any delay would lead to serious harm or death. If a competent young person refuses treatment it is probable that the administration of even life-saving treatment would be unlawful. The Scottish courts have not, however, made a definitive ruling on this matter. Doctors are therefore advised that, because of the significance of pre-empting the courts' views, emergency life-saving treatment should be given and an application made to a court for its determination of the issues as a matter of urgency. In all cases of refusal of treatment, if time permits there should be discussion with the family and attempts at resolution. Legal advice should be sought.[11]

3.2 Consent from competent young people

As in England, Wales and Northern Ireland, the consent of parents is not always needed before treating children and young people. In Scotland the age of majority is 18[12] but young people can make many legally binding decisions before that age. The presumption that a person can make most decisions, including whether to consent to medical treatment, arises at the age of 16. It is provided for by statute, which states that "a person of or over the age of 16 years shall have legal capacity to enter into any transaction".[13] While this may not immediately appear to have much to do with medical treatment, transaction "means a transaction having legal effect and includes ... the giving by a person of any consent having legal effect".[14] Since consent to medical treatment can have the legal effect of preventing an action for assault, medical treatment is covered by this law.

There is no statutory definition of competence in relation to these provisions, and patients between 16 and 18 should be presumed competent to give consent, as adults are. This is the case even if, for example, the proposed medical intervention is not for the patient's therapeutic benefit, such as tissue or organ donation.[15]

Since 1991 there has also been statutory provision for consent to medical treatment by those under 16.

> *A person under the age of 16 years shall have legal capacity to consent on his own behalf to any surgical, medical or dental procedure or treatment where, in the opinion of a qualified medical practitioner attending him, he is capable of understanding the nature and possible consequences of the procedure or treatment.*[16]

At the time of writing, only one reported case (*Houston, applicant*) had dealt with the interpretation of this section.[17] The implications of the case in respect of refusal of consent are considered below.

3.2.1 Competence

The Age of Legal Capacity (Scotland) Act states that the assessment of a child's understanding is to be made by "a qualified medical practitioner attending the child".[18] It is doubtful that the legislators intended this to exclude the possibility of health professionals other than doctors judging competence, for example dentists when dental treatment is at issue. It has been suggested that the decision to refer to "qualified" rather than "registered" medical practitioners in the Act, which is the term generally used in statutes such as the Abortion Act 1967, means that any health professional qualified to perform the treatment or procedure can make the assessment of the child's understanding. Qualified might then be read in relation to the health professional's qualification to perform the procedure or treatment rather than qualified to assess understanding.[19] The statute certainly does not have an express requirement that the medical practitioner have any specific training or expertise in assessment of understanding nor, more particularly, assessment of understanding in children, although this may be desirable. Practical aspects of the assessment of competence are discussed in chapter 5.

The Act says that children are competent to make decisions when they satisfy a medical practitioner of their understanding. The decision of the qualified medical practitioner on this matter was intended to be final. In drafting its Bill, the Scottish Law Commission considered a number of options, one of which was for doctors to provide treatment to those under 16 where the child "was capable" of understanding the nature and consequences of proposed treatment. This approach was rejected since it would require the doctor to determine as a matter of fact rather than opinion whether the child was competent. It was thought to "give little protection to doctors and might make them reluctant to give treatment on the basis of a young person's own consent except in the most obvious and uncontroversial cases".[20] Instead, the legislation makes clear that doctors may rely on consent from somebody who *in their opinion* is capable of understanding the nature and possible consequences of the proposed treatment.

The law gives no guidance on situations where there is disagreement between medical practitioners caring for a child. In contrast, the Adults with Incapacity (Scotland) Act provides that it is the medical practitioner with *primary responsibility* for the care of the adult who is to certify incompetence and who has authority either to provide treatment him or herself, or instruct others to do so.[21] This is absent from the legislation dealing with children. Whilst even this may cause some difficulties in interpretation, it does provide a hierarchical structure for resolving differences of opinion that is absent from the previous legislation. If there is disagreement amongst health professionals caring for children, it may be necessary to seek legal advice about the authority to proceed.

Unlike the law in England, Wales and Northern Ireland, which is commonly believed to exclude non-therapeutic procedures from the scope of competent young people's consent,[22] nothing in Scottish law prevents competent young people, including those under 16, from giving valid consent to non-therapeutic procedures, for example tissue donation.[23] Nevertheless, readers are advised to note the discussion in chapter 8 regarding reservations about tissue donation and, in particular, the BMA's opposition to minors donating whole organs or non-regenerative tissue. As discussed above, the medical practitioner is invited to form an opinion about the child's understanding, not whether the proposed intervention is in the child's interests. The statute does not elaborate on the kind of ability the young person needs, nor whether his or her choice must be wise, although the High Court in England has been clear that the test is whether the patient under 16 is capable of making a choice, not whether it is a wise choice.[24]

3.2.2 Confidentiality

Where a competent young person gives consent to medical treatment, the permission of parents is not legally necessary. Indeed, treatment may proceed without the parents' knowledge or against their wishes. Whilst the question of confidentiality is not directly addressed in Scottish statute, it is generally understood that all competent patients are owed the same duty of confidentiality. This approach is shown in the guidance of professional and regulatory bodies, which give adults and children the same rights to confidentiality (see chapter 4).[25] This is also the view taken in advice issued in 1992, in a letter from the National Health Service Executive in Scotland, which states that:

> *In the majority of cases children will be accompanied by their parents during consultations. Where exceptionally a child is seen alone, efforts should be made to persuade the child that his or her parents should be informed except in circumstances where it is clearly not in the best interests of the child to do so. However, if a child capable of understanding the nature and consequences of the treatment refuses to allow parent(s) or guardian(s) to be informed, the doctor should respect the rules of professional confidentiality.*[26]

It should be noted that in Scotland parents have a statutory right and responsibility to provide direction and guidance to their children because of provisions in the Children (Scotland) Act. The right and responsibility to give direction last until the child is 16[27] but the responsibility to give guidance lasts until the young person is 18.[28] It has been suggested that in order to be able to give guidance and direction it might be considered necessary for parents to be informed of important matters affecting the child, such as controversial medical treatment.

> *... [I]t is precisely where medical treatment is not unarguably in the child's best interests that parents should have the right to be informed and be able to advise their children before they embark on a course of action which they may later regret.*[29]

Examples such as obtaining contraceptives, having a termination of pregnancy and donating non-regenerative tissue were suggested (see also chapter 8).

Requiring confidentiality to be breached, however, so that parents can give guidance even if they have no right to override the child's decision would represent a serious disincentive to children to seek medical advice and treatment. Furthermore, it is precisely in connection with treatments that may be seen as controversial that young people are most likely to want their confidentiality maintained. It may be that any conflict between a child's right to confidentiality and the parental right to give direction and guidance can be resolved by the fact that parental direction and guidance must be appropriate to the stage of development of the child. Direction and guidance are also limited to what is practicable and in the best interests of the child. Whether and in what circumstances parents have a right to be informed to fulfil these statutory responsibilities may perhaps be regarded as legally uncertain.[30] Nevertheless, the BMA recognises the significance of a decision to breach the confidentiality of a young person and advises doctors to adopt the same approach to confidentiality in Scotland as in other UK jurisdictions (see chapter 4).

3.2.3 People over 16

When people reach the age of 16 they are presumed to be competent to make decisions about their medical care, although competence may be affected by illness or injury. If this is the case, parents do not have an automatic right to make decisions on their child's behalf. Their rights to act as their child's legal representatives cease when the young person reaches 16.[31]

The care of people over 16 years of age who cannot make decisions about medical treatment is governed by the Adults with Incapacity (Scotland) Act. The Act gives authority to the doctor with primary responsibility for caring for patients who lack competence to do what is reasonable in the circumstances to safeguard or promote their physical or mental health. The doctor must certify that, for a specified time period (which cannot be longer than one year), the patient is not capable of making his or her own decisions. The Act contains rules governing the criteria to be taken into account, consultations that should take place and the methods of appealing against decisions. The Act leaves the option for ministers to define specific treatments that should be handled outwith this regime. The Act says that relatives should be consulted, but they can only make a decision on behalf of a person over 16 who lacks competence if they have been appointed by the patient as a proxy decision maker (a welfare guardian). Conditions apply for the exercise of decision making powers both by medical practitioners and by welfare guardians. In the event of disagreement or uncertainty, legal advice should be sought.

3.2.4 Refusal by competent young people

As discussed in chapter 2, at its time the *Gillick* case was presumed to give competent young people the right to refuse as well as consent to medical treatment, but subsequent case law has not borne out this interpretation. It seems that Scots law, however, is developing differently. There has been only one reported case that concerned refusal of treatment and the scope of the medical treatment provisions of the Age of Legal Capacity (Scotland) Act.[32]

The Houston case

An application was made to Glasgow Sheriff Court for formal detention of a 15-year-old under the Mental Health (Scotland) Act 1984. The patient had been diagnosed as having symptoms of a psychotic illness. Two consultant psychiatrists believed that his condition fell within the definition of a mental disorder and that it was of a nature and degree that made it appropriate for him to receive treatment in hospital. They were also of the opinion that it was necessary for his health and safety that he should receive medical treatment in hospital.

He refused treatment, however, and also refused to remain in hospital. The doctors believed that he was capable of understanding the nature and possible consequences of treatment and was therefore legally competent to make decisions on these matters. The doctors also believed that the right to consent carried with it the right to refuse, and therefore treatment would only be lawful if it fell within the scope of mental health legislation.

His mother was prepared to give consent to his treatment and detention in hospital and it was argued on her behalf that, since she was prepared to consent, the proposed order was unnecessary. In determining the case, the Sheriff recognised that there is a stigma associated with detention under the mental health legislation and that this should be avoided by treating without a detention order if possible.

Despite expressing some reservations about whether the

---

mother's consent was valid, the Sheriff tended to the view that the decision of a competent young person could not be overruled by a parent. He concluded that logic demanded that when a young person was declared competent, the young person's decision took precedence over that of a parent. Furthermore, he considered that the Age of Legal Capacity (Scotland) Act covered refusal as well as consent to treatment.

In the circumstances, the Sheriff granted the detention order with the observation that, despite the stigma, the patient's serious illness and its treatment were the paramount considerations.

Houston, applicant

If the Sheriff's views reflect a correct interpretation of the law, once children of any age are judged competent they can consent to or refuse treatment. This would seem to follow logic and the majority of commentators appear to support this position.[33] It is also supported in National Health Service guidance published shortly after the commencement of the Age of Legal Capacity (Scotland) Act, which advises that if, after careful explanation of the consequences of failure to treat, "the patient then refuses to agree, and he or she is competent, the refusal must be respected. The doctor should record this in the clinical notes and where possible have it witnessed".[34]

In this case, however, the issue of whether the Sheriff had the power to override the refusal of a competent young person was actually avoided because there was an alternative way of dealing with the case and treatment was given under mental health legislation. A case concerning proposed treatment falling outwith the provisions of mental health legislation has yet to be decided.

3.2.5 A statutory right to refuse

The Children (Scotland) Act gives competent young people the right to refuse to submit to medical or psychiatric examination or other assessment that has been directed by the court or a children's hearing for the purpose of supervision requirement, assessment, protection or place of safety order.[35] This part of the Act is concerned with children's hearings and the promotion of children's welfare by local authorities, and does not refer to parental rights and responsibilities or orders made under other sections of the Act.[36] The statutory right to refuse mirrors provisions in the English legislation, which, as chapter 2 has discussed, can be overridden by a court,[37] although this has been the subject of perceptive criticism in England.[38] In view of this criticism and the generally more empowering approach of Scots law towards young people it is thought unlikely that the Scottish courts would follow suit.

3.2.6 Comment on the law

As discussed in chapter 2, the BMA's view is that there is a need for greater clarity about when it is legally permissible to override a young person's wishes and when it is not. The legal issues could be clarified by the courts or statute, and would be an appropriate subject for consideration by the Scottish Law Commission. Meanwhile, this book is the Association's attempt to provide as much guidance as it is presently possible to do and doctors are advised to approach their lawyers if there is doubt.

3.3 Consent from parents and people with parental responsibility

3.3.1 Parental responsibilities

A person who has parental responsibility for a child may, in law, consent to treatment on that child's behalf, at least as long as the child is unable to make such decisions. The rules about parental responsibility are described below, but if there is any doubt about whether the person giving consent is lawfully entitled to do so, doctors should seek further advice.

Parental responsibilities include safeguarding and promoting the child's health, welfare and development, providing direction and guidance to the child in a manner appropriate to the stage of the child's development and acting as the child's legal representative.[39] Parental rights are accorded to enable parental responsibilities to be carried out. All parental rights end when the young person is 16, although some may be lost before this if the child attains legal capacity to act on his or her own behalf. The parental responsibility to provide guidance lasts until the young person is 18.

A child's biological parents are the child's legal parents, unless he or she has been adopted or was born as the result of some methods of assisted reproduction. Where the child has been adopted, the adopters are the child's legal parents. Where the child has been born as a result of assisted reproduction, there are rules under the Human Fertilisation and Embryology Act 1990 that determine the child's legal parentage.

Not all parents have parental responsibilities and rights. Both parents have parental responsibilities and rights if they were married at the time of the child's conception, or birth, or at some time after the child's birth.[40] These are not lost if they divorce.

If the parents have never married, only the mother automatically has parental responsibilities and rights. The father may acquire these through a voluntary parental responsibility agreement with the mother made in a prescribed form and registered in the Books of Council and Session.[41] Alternatively fathers may apply to the Sheriff Court or Court of Session for an order to give them parental responsibilities and rights. In this case, the child's welfare is the paramount consideration and the court will only make such an order if satisfied that it is in the best interests of the child. The issue of the parental responsibilities and rights of unmarried fathers is currently under review in Scotland because of concerns that the current provisions are in breach of international obligations.[42] The possible implications of the Human Rights Act on the rights of fathers is discussed in section 2.3. The BMA will put information about any changes to the rules on its website.

People other than a child's biological parents can acquire parental responsibilities and rights by being appointed as guardians (the appointment taking effect on the death of the parents)[43] or on the order of a court.[44] For example, a local authority may acquire parental responsibility by obtaining a parental responsibilities order.[45]

3.3.2 Limits on parental rights

Where a competent young person refuses treatment

Parents have a range of rights to enable them to carry out their parental responsibilities towards their children, including the right to act as the child's legal representative. This right enables parents to consent to treatment on behalf of children who are obviously unable to give consent. Before the Age of Legal Capacity (Scotland) Act came into force, a case with very similar facts to those in *Houston, applicant* was heard in the Sheriff Court.[46]

The case of V v F

A mental health officer applied to have a 15-year-old mentally ill patient compulsorily detained under section 18 of the Mental Health (Scotland) Act. The patient opposed the application on the grounds that it was not necessary for her health or safety or for the protection of other people.

The evidence presented to the court was that she was prepared to consent to taking prescribed treatment but that she was not always prepared to stay in the hospital and at times was in danger of harming herself. On these occasions she required to be restrained.

Her parents were prepared to consent on their daughter's behalf to her medical treatment and to any necessary restraint should she seek to leave the hospital or harm herself.

The Sheriff concluded that the parents were able to consent on behalf of their daughter and therefore that it was unnecessary to make a detention order.

V v F

In reaching his conclusion, the Sheriff referred to the powers that parents had as curators of their minor children and to the case of *Gillick*. He held that it was the curators' responsibility and duty to care for their children and to make decisions on their behalf when they could not do so themselves. Parents are no longer termed curators of their children but instead are referred to as "guardians". It is arguable, however, that they perform the same function. Following this reasoning, it has been suggested that parents can give consent to treatment for competent children. This argument is weakened by the fact that in *V v F* no explicit finding was made of the patient's own ability to consent to or refuse treatment. Although the Sheriff expressed little doubt that she understood the evidence and in general terms the requirements of the proposed order, he also described her as vulnerable and ill. It may be that *V v F* is best seen as an example of parents giving consent on behalf of an incapable child, rather than as an example of parents being able to override the decision of a competent young person.[47]

The later case of *Houston, applicant* provides stronger support for the view that once a young person has legal capacity, parents lose any right to override their child's decision. It is arguable that the Sheriff's remarks are not binding but only passing comments (*obiter dicta*), since he expressed doubt about the validity of the mother's consent, which was described as being "far from unqualified or clear". Nevertheless, the provisions of the Children (Scotland) Act, enacted after *V v F*, also seem to support the idea that parents cannot override the decision of a child with legal capacity. It states that a parent can only act as the child's legal representative, for example by giving consent to medical treatment, "where the child is incapable of so acting or consenting on his own behalf".[48] The position of parents whose competent child makes a valid decision is arguably, therefore, outwith the statutory provisions. It would seem that parents cannot override their competent child's decisions[49] although the matter has yet to be settled authoritatively.

The child's best interests

Although presumed to be the appropriate decision makers for children unable to decide themselves, parents' powers to determine whether a treatment goes ahead are limited and parents must act in their child's best interests.

In the case described below, the parents' refusal to allow their child to be given blood products was regarded as amounting to wilful neglect and lack of parental care in legal proceedings, despite the fact that the parents believed they were acting in the best interests of the child.[50] (Similar issues are raised in the English case *Re C (A Child) (HIV Testing)* discussed in sections 1.4.5 and 2.3.2.)

Case of Finlayson

The child, whose name was not disclosed, was found to suffer from severe haemophilia when he had an operation at six months of age. His parents were told of the nature of the condition and that their child should be brought in for treatment whenever and as soon as bleeding occurred.

The parents were devastated about their child's illness and were also concerned at the possibility that he might contract AIDS through blood transfusions. They favoured alternative medicine and homoeopathic remedies. Nevertheless, the parents initially took the child to a haemophilia centre for review every six months. During this time, there were a few occasions in which the parents noticed signs of bleeding on the child with bruising, swelling and soreness. They gave him mild analgesics, comforted him and he appeared to get better. They did not tell the haemophilia centre about these episodes.

When the child was two, he had a significant bleed in his right knee. He was treated at the centre with cryoprecipitate. The parents did not want him treated with Factor VIII. Due to an administrative error, he was then not seen at the centre for four years, during which time he had a number of bleeds after falls. His parents treated him with herbal remedies. When the child was invited to attend the haemophilia centre again, it was found that his right knee had been subject to chronic bleeding that had been going on for some time. As a result, the bones in his knee were enlarged and he limped. The damage to the knee was largely permanent.

The parents were reluctant to agree to the proposed treatment, and in particular to the use of blood products. The parents wished to have their child treated by a local GP who also used homoeopathic remedies and to have resort to the haemophilia centre and blood products only in an emergency. They reserved to themselves the right to decide what was an emergency. They did not accept that there was a high risk that their child would end up with serious damage if untreated with Factor VIII.

The doctor at the centre contacted social services and, after the child missed follow up appointments, a reporter to the children's hearing system was involved to investigate whether the child was in need of compulsory measures of care, such as a supervision requirement with a condition requiring the child to attend for medical examination or treatment. [A description of the role of the reporter is given in section 3.5.1 below.]

The reporter decided that grounds for referral to a children's hearing were satisfied but the parents disagreed. The matter was therefore taken to the Sheriff Court to determine whether the grounds for referral were indeed satisfied.

The Sheriff held that in spite of the fact that the parents were loving and concerned with the health of the child, their refusal to consent to conventional treatment constituted wilful neglect and lack of parental care likely to cause the child unnecessary suffering or serious impairment to his health or development. The Sheriff reached this conclusion based on what a "reasonable person" would consider acceptable conduct. The grounds for referral were established and the case was referred to a children's hearing for its decision on how to proceed.

Finlayson, applicant

This case illustrates very clearly the potential for disagreement over how a child's welfare is best protected. Cases like this are, fortunately, uncommon, and doctors can usually rely on parents' judgments about what is in their young child's best interests. Support for this presumption that parents make decisions is seen in the European Convention on Human Rights[51] and the Children (Scotland) Act. Accordingly, a court or children's hearing invited to override the wishes of parents must do so extremely cautiously in cases where the child cannot express his or her own views.

There are no reported Scottish cases of courts being asked to intervene because parents ask for treatment that the health team believe is inappropriate. In the absence of such case law, reference may be made to the approach of the High Court in England, which, although not binding, may be persuasive (see chapter 2). Where continued treatment is not in a child's best interests, the courts have allowed the health team to withdraw or withhold treatment from children against the parents' wishes. For an example of such a case, see the description of *Re C (A Minor) (Medical Treatment)* in section 2.3.2.

Chapter 2 also describes a controversial case in which the court upheld the refusal of parents to give consent to a life-saving liver transplant for their baby boy (see *Re T (A Minor) (Wardship: Medical Treatment)*, section 2.3.2). Whether the Scottish courts would have approached the facts of this case in the same way is of course a matter of speculation. Nevertheless, in any jurisdiction, concerns over the integrity of families and respect for their decisions must be weighed along with the needs of the individual child and there can be no simple formula to resolve such issues.

3.4 Consent from carers

As in England, Wales and Northern Ireland, any person who has care of a child may do "what is reasonable in all the circumstances of the case for the purpose of safeguarding or promoting the child's welfare".[52] This could include giving consent to medical treatment. Parents are also entitled to authorise another person to take over particular responsibilities.[53] This might be because parents have arranged for somebody else to look after their child while they are away. It is unlikely to be reasonable for a non-parent to give consent if he or she knows that the child's parents are likely to object, and treatment should only be given in such circumstances if the situation is an emergency and delay would lead to serious harm or death. If a carer brings a child for treatment, steps should be taken to ascertain the parents' views, and if there is doubt about authority to proceed, doctors should seek legal advice.

3.5 Consent from the courts and children's hearings

The courts have the power to give consent to treatment on behalf of a person under 16 where the child is not competent to give valid consent for him or herself. It is unclear whether a court may override the decision of a child where the medical practitioner believes the child is competent, although it is thought that this is unlikely (see sections 3.2.5 and 3.5.2). This issue may need to be resolved by a test case or legislation. If in doubt, doctors should approach their lawyers for advice.

3.5.1 Mechanisms for involvement

Section 3.5.3 suggests circumstances in which legal proceedings may be necessary. If any of these situations arise, doctors should seek legal advice. If advice suggests that proceedings are necessary, there are various mechanisms that can be invoked. The courts are available at all hours for matters requiring urgent attention. Both the Sheriff Court and the Court of Session can make medical treatment decisions, and can appoint a curator *ad litem* whose duty it is to safeguard the interests of the child by ensuring that the case is conducted properly on the child's behalf.[54] Outside normal office hours, contact should be made, normally by a lawyer, with the local

Sheriff Court or alternatively with the Keeper's Office for cases being brought to the Court of Session. The urgency of the situation will be assessed and, if appropriate, a Sheriff or Judge Depute contacted. The matter may be dealt with over the telephone, or the Sheriff or Judge Depute may direct attendance at his or her home. Lawyers may therefore find it prudent to have a medical expert available to speak to the Sheriff or Judge Depute in such circumstances.

Welfare and proportionality

When a court determines any matter relating to parental responsibilities and rights, it is required by law to have the child's welfare as the paramount consideration and not to make any order unless satisfied that to do so would be better than making none at all. It is also required to comply with the Human Rights Act, and apply the rights and freedoms of the European Convention on Human Rights.[55] The court must, so far as practicable, give the child the opportunity to express views and, having regard to age and maturity, have regard to those views.[56]

Children (Scotland) Act

The most likely form of proceeding is to seek an order concerning parental rights and responsibilities under the Children (Scotland) Act. The court can invoke statutory provisions to authorise or prohibit steps taken in the exercise of parental responsibility in relation to medical treatment. It can make a specific issue order ("an order regulating any specific question which has arisen or may arise" in connection with parental responsibilities, parental rights or guardianship),[57] or a prohibited steps order ("an interdict prohibiting the taking of any step of a kind specified in the interdict in the fulfilment of parental responsibilities or the exercise of parental rights relating to a child").[58]

The inherent jurisdiction

In addition to specific legislation giving the courts power, the Court of Session has an ancient, non-statutory (inherent) jurisdiction. The *parens patriae* jurisdiction gives the Court of Session the power to give consent to or refuse medical treatment for children and incapacitated adults. This provision is rarely invoked for people under 16 because of the wide powers of the courts under the Children (Scotland) Act.[59] The courts have held that the jurisdiction entitles the courts to authorise the withdrawal of treatment from a patient for whom continued treatment did not provide a benefit, although because opinions may vary about what is a "benefit" doctors' views will be sought (see chapter 6).[60] Consideration must also be given to patients' rights under the Human Rights Act. The *parens patriae* jurisdiction's use may diminish for adult patients in the future following the introduction of a comprehensive proxy decision making procedures in the Adults with Incapacity (Scotland) Act. Decisions made under this jurisdiction may still be necessary where withdrawing or withholding treatment is contemplated, however, since the Adults with Incapacity (Scotland) Act covers only the provision of treatment. Proposed provisions relating to withdrawal of treatment were not enacted.

The children's hearing system

An alternative procedure to protect the health and welfare of children is to go through the children's hearing system. This system is unique to Scotland in the United Kingdom. It was developed to respond to children in need of help and is based on the view that children who commit offences are as likely to need support as children who are victims of offences. It is concerned with a broad spectrum of issues concerning the welfare of children and has wide ranging powers.

Anyone who believes that a child requires compulsory measures of supervision (for example a social worker, policeman or doctor) may contact a reporter.[61] A court may also refer a child to a reporter.[62] The reporter investigates and decides whether a ground for referral to a children's hearing is established. There are several potential grounds for referral and the most relevant here is that the child is likely either to suffer unnecessarily or to suffer serious impairment in his or her health or development, due to lack of parental care.[63] These matters are determined objectively so that a finding of lack of parental care can be established even where parents are deeply concerned with the welfare of their child and are providing what they consider to be the best care for him or her (see section 3.3.2).

If a ground for referral is established, a hearing will be convened. If there is agreement by the relevant people, including the competent young person and his or her parents, the hearing can go on to decide how the issue should be dealt with and make an appropriate order. If they do not accept the ground for referral, the case must be sent to a Sheriff Court for determination. Only if the Sheriff decides that the ground for referral is made out can the case be returned to the children's hearing for it to deal with it. Otherwise the Sheriff will dismiss the application.

A children's hearing can deal with cases in a number of ways, including making a supervision order with conditions attached. Such conditions could include requiring the attendance of the child for medical examination or treatment.

Legal advice

Whether it is more appropriate to pursue a case through the children's hearing system or through proceedings in the Sheriff Court or Court of Session depends on the facts of the case. Since a court can refer a case to a reporter in the course of proceedings concerning parental responsibilities and rights, it may be that cases would be better started in this forum. Court proceedings may also be more appropriate where the case concerns a one-off treatment or a matter that requires to be decided quickly. It is probably also the only proper form of proceeding where there is any dispute over the child's own ability to consent to treatment. Legal advice and advice from social services should be sought on the most appropriate proceedings, where these are thought necessary.

3.5.2 Limits on the powers of courts and children's hearings

It is unclear whether the courts have the power to override the decision of a competent young person. It has been suggested that a court could override the decision of a competent young person since it has the right to make an order "in relation to (a) parental responsibilities and (b) parental rights" until a child is 16.[64] When making such an order, the court must have the welfare of the child as the paramount consideration. Therefore it has been argued that if the decision by the young person is not considered to be in his or her best interests, the court could override it.[65]

Giving consent to medical treatment for a child is undoubtedly an aspect of the exercise of parental responsibilities and rights. It is hard to see, however, why a court should be able to make an order in respect of a parental responsibility or right that a parent cannot. Courts generally exercise parental rights where there is no parent able and willing to do so in an appropriate manner, not where the parental right has effectively ceased to exist. It has therefore been argued that once a young person is competent to make the decision in question, the matter in hand is no longer one of parental responsibilities and rights and therefore any applications for the court to overrule a competent decision should be dismissed.[66]

These considerations strongly suggest that a court cannot override a competent child's decision in the interests of that child, any more than it could override the decision of a competent adult in that adult's best interests (although there may be other reasons why treatment decisions might be overridden, such as the protection of others). Nevertheless, there is no definitive ruling on this matter and whether a court can override a competent child's refusal of treatment is perhaps most accurately described as uncertain.

In this regard, it is worth remembering that the English cases on refusal of consent after *Gillick* provoked considerable surprise among commentators and the approach of Scottish courts may prove to be equally unpredictable. Opinions differ sharply about whether it is appropriate to allow competent young people to make decisions that may cause them to suffer serious, irreversible harm. There may be less scope for broad interpretation of the statutes in Scotland than in other parts of the UK, but the Scottish judiciary may well be as anxious to prevent avoidable harm to children and young people as their English counterparts.[67] Even despite advice from the NHS that refusal of consent by competent young people under 16 must be respected,[68] doctors are urged to be cautious where refusal has serious implications for the patient's health. Where there is controversy, doctors should approach their lawyers for advice about whether the case should be brought before a court.

3.5.3 *When to go to court*

Whilst it is neither helpful nor desirable to draw up a definitive list of situations that should be taken to court, some generalisations can be made to help doctors to identify when they should seek legal advice.

Legal advice should be sought when:

- agreement over how to proceed cannot be reached (for example where consent is refused by the holders of parental responsibility);
- a competent young person refuses invasive treatment;

- administering treatment against the wishes of a competent young person would require the use of restraint or force;
- it is not clear whether the people with parental responsibility are acting in the best interests of the child;
- the proposed care is beyond the scope of parental consent because it is controversial or non-therapeutic (for example sterilisation, organ donation and circumcision if parents disagree);
- the courts require legal review of the decision;
- the treatment requires detention outwith the provisions of mental health legislation;
- the people with parental responsibility lack the competence to make the decision; or
- the proposed course of action might breach a person's Convention rights.

The role of the court is to declare whether the proposed course of action is lawful, and to do so with regard to the best interests of the child in question. It has been held in the English courts that the courts do not have the power to require a doctor to treat (see section 2.5.3). There is no reason to suppose that the Scottish courts would take a different view. Thus, whilst the authorisation of a court tells doctors that treatment is lawful, it does not mean that treatment must definitely go ahead. Doctors must still assess whether treatment is appropriate and whether it is in the child's best interests (see chapter 1).

The alternative mechanism of children's hearings may also be appropriate in certain circumstances.

3.6 Summary

Decisions about the medical treatment of children should ideally be taken by children together with their parents.

In Scotland treatment may be given to a person under 16 provided that there is valid consent from:

- a competent child;
- a person or local authority with parental responsibility;
- a court; or
- a person caring for a child but only if the proposed procedure is reasonable in all the circumstances to safeguard the child's health, development and welfare.

It is important to note, however, that if a competent child refuses consent to treatment, from current case law and statute it seems likely that this refusal of consent cannot be overridden by any other person, a carer or a court. This matter is not beyond doubt and legal advice should be sought where such situations arise.

Consent does not necessarily mean that treatment must be given and the Scottish Law Commission has stressed that "the fact that legally effective consent is given to treatment does not oblige a doctor to proceed with that treatment".[69] Doctors have legal and ethical obligations over and above the requirement to obtain valid consent, and should not proceed if, in their clinical judgment, giving treatment is inappropriate. At the core of these obligations is respect for human rights.

Whoever gives consent for the treatment, the child's wishes are an essential part of assessing what is in his or her best interests. Sustained wishes should not be overridden lightly, and all children should be offered the opportunity for their views to be heard and given due consideration.

Where there is no one available who can give a valid consent it is lawful for doctors to proceed with treatment immediately necessary to preserve life, health or wellbeing until it is possible to seek consent from the appropriate person.[70] If there is an emergency and any delay would lead to serious harm or death, life-saving treatment may be given against the wishes of an incompetent child or his or her parents. In the absence of a clear ruling from the Scottish courts as to whether a competent child may refuse life-saving treatment the BMA advises that emergency life-saving treatment should be given and an application made to a court as a matter of urgency.

References

1 The legal concepts of pupils and minors derived from Roman law have not disappeared entirely but are not relevant to the issues considered in this document.

2 The Scottish Executive has stated that implementation of the Adults with Incapacity (Scotland) Act 2000 will commence in April 2001 and be completed in April 2002. Additional regulations and codes of practice to implement the Act will also be issued.

3 Readers are advised to check the BMA's website for information about any recent developments.

4 Scottish Law Commission. *Report on the legal capacity and responsibility of minors and pupils no 110*. Edinburgh: SLC, 1987.

5 Convention for the Protection of Human Rights and Fundamental Freedoms (4. ix. 1950; TS 71; Cmnd 8969).

6 Scotland Act 1998 s29.

7 Scotland Act 1998 s57(2).

8 Procedures for asserting rights under the Human Rights Act 1998 and Scotland Act 1998 are outwith the scope of this document. For further discussion, see Scottish Office. *Human rights: the European Convention on Human Rights, the Scotland Act* and the *Human Rights Act*. Edinburgh: Scottish Office, 1999; Scottish Human Rights Centre. *Human Rights and the Scottish Parliament*. Glasgow: SHRC, 1998; Wadham J, Mountfield H. *Blackstone's guide to the Human Rights Act 1998*. London: Blackstone Press, 1999.

9 Houston, applicant 1996 SCLR 943, (1996) 32 BMLR 93. Children (Scotland) Act 1995 s15(5)(b) and 90.

10 Scottish Law Commission. *Report on the legal capacity and responsibility of minors and pupils no 110*. Edinburgh: SLC, 1987: paras 3.79 and 3.80; National Health Service in Scotland Management Executive. *A guide to consent to examination, investigation, treatment or operation*. Edinburgh: NHS in Scotland Management Executive, 1992: ch 2, para 16. See also the English case Re F (Mental Patient: Sterilisation) [1990] 2 AC 1, [1989] 2 WLR 1025, [1989] 2 All ER 545, [1989] 2 FLR 376, HL.

11 Two English cases involving Jehovah's Witness children have suggested that the approval of a court should be sought before the administration of treatment where parents and children refuse. Re O (A Minor) (Medical Treatment) [1993] 2 FLR 149, [1993] 1 FCR 925, [1993] 4 Med LR 272; Re S (A Minor) (Medical Treatment) [1993] 1 FLR 377, [1993] Fam Law 215.

12 Age of Majority (Scotland) Act 1969 s1.

13 Age of Legal Capacity (Scotland) Act 1991 s1(1)(b). There are provisions designed to protect children from having made unwise choices by allowing them to set aside prejudicial transactions, under certain conditions, until they have reached the age of 21. Consent to medical, dental or surgical treatment cannot be set aside, however. Age of Legal Capacity (Scotland) Act 1991 s3(3)(e).

14 Age of Legal Capacity (Scotland) Act 1991 s9.

15 The Scottish Law Commission expressly took this possibility into account in drafting its Bill. Scottish Law Commission. *Report on the legal capacity and responsibility of minors and pupils no 110*. Edinburgh: SLC, 1987: para 3.76. This may be contrasted with the view of Lord Donaldson in Re W (A Minor) (Medical Treatment: Court's Jurisdiction) [1993] Fam 64, [1992] 3 WLR 758, [1992] 4 All ER 627, CA that the corresponding English provision would not permit 16 to 18 year olds to consent to organ or blood donation since these were not treatments.

16 Age of Legal Capacity (Scotland) Act 1991 s2(4).

17 Houston, applicant 1996 SCLR 943, (1996) 32 BMLR 93.

18 Age of Legal Capacity (Scotland) Act 1991 s2(4).

19 Wilkinson AB, Norrie KMcK. *The law relating to parent and child in Scotland*, 2nd edition. Edinburgh: W Green, 1999: para 15.09: 480.

20 Scottish Law Commission. *Report on the legal capacity and responsibility of minors and pupils no 110*. Edinburgh: SLC, 1987: para 3.73.

21 Adults with Incapacity (Scotland) Act 2000 s47.

22 Montgomery J. *Health care law*. Oxford: Oxford University Press, 1997: 283.

23 Scottish Law Commission. *Report on the legal capacity and responsibility of minors and pupils no 110*. Edinburgh: SLC, 1987: paras 3.76—3.78.

24 South Glamorgan CC v B, sub nom South Glamorgan CC v W and B [1993] FLR 574, [1993] 1 FCR 626, [1993] Fam Law 398.

25 General Medical Council. *Confidentiality: protecting and providing information*. London: GMC, 2000.

26 National Health Service in Scotland Management Executive. *A guide to consent to examination, investigation, treatment or operation*. Edinburgh: NHS in Scotland Management Executive, 1992: ch 2, para 10.

27 Children (Scotland) Act 1995 s1(1)(b)(i), 1(2)(a) and 2(7).

28 Children (Scotland) Act 1995 s1(1)(b)(ii) and 1(2)(b).

29 Thomson JM. *Family law in Scotland*, 3rd edition. Edinburgh: Butterworths/Law

Society of Scotland, 1996: 209.

30 As Norrie puts it, a right to advise does not include the right to be consulted in all cases. Norrie KMcK. *Family planning and the law*. Aldershot: Dartmouth, 1991: 102—5.

31 Children (Scotland) Act 1995 s1(1)(b)(ii) and 1(2)(b).

32 Houston, applicant 1996 SCLR 943, (1996) 32 BMLR 93.

33 Thomson JM. *Family law in Scotland*, 3rd edition. Edinburgh: Butterworths/Law Society of Scotland, 1996: 167—8; Wilkinson AB, Norrie KMcK. *The law relating to parent and child in Scotland*, 2nd edition. Edinburgh: W Green, 1999; Sutherland EE. *Child and family law*. Edinburgh: T & T Clark, 1999: para 3.71.

34 National Health Service in Scotland Management Executive. *A guide to consent to examination, investigation, treatment or operation*. Edinburgh: NHS in Scotland Management Executive, 1992: ch 2, para 14.

35 Children (Scotland) Act 1995 s90.

36 It does cover parental responsibilities transferred to a local authority under the Children (Scotland) Act 1995 s86.

37 South Glamorgan CC v B, sub nom South Glamorgan CC v W and B [1993] FLR 574, [1993] 1 FCR 626, [1993] Fam Law 398.

38 Kennedy I, Grubb A, eds. *Principles of Medical Law*. Oxford: University Press, 1998.

39 Children (Scotland) Act 1995 s1(1).

40 Children (Scotland) Act 1995 s3(1)(a) and (b).

41 Children (Scotland) Act 1995 s4.

42 See for example Norrie KMcK. *Children (Scotland) Act 1995*. Edinburgh: W Green, 1995.

43 Children (Scotland) Act 1995 s7.

44 Children (Scotland) Act 1995 s11(3)(a).

45 Children (Scotland) Act 1995 s86.

46 V v F 1991 SCLR 225.

47 One commentator at least suggests that *V v F* and *Houston, applicant* represent two conflicting lines of authority. Grubb A. Commentary on Houston, applicant. *Medical Law Review* 1997;5:237—9.

48 Children (Scotland) Act 1995 s15(5)(b).

49 Norrie KMcK. *Children (Scotland) Act 1995*. Edinburgh: W Green, 1995: paras 36—43.

50 Finlayson, applicant, sub nom Finlayson v I 1989 SCLR 601.

51 Convention for the Protection of Human Rights and Fundamental Freedoms (4. ix. 1950; TS 71; Cmnd 8969).

52 Children (Scotland) Act 1995 s5(1).

53 Children (Scotland) Act 1995 s3(5).

54 Age of Legal Capacity (Scotland) Act 1991 s1(3)(f)(ii).

55 Convention for the Protection of Human Rights and Fundamental Freedoms (4. ix. 1950; TS 71; Cmnd 8969).

56 Children (Scotland) Act 1995 s11(7).

57 Children (Scotland) Act 1995 s11(2)(e).

58 Children (Scotland) Act 1995 s11(7)(f).

59 See also Wilkinson AB, Norrie KMcK. *The law relating to parent and child in Scotland*, 2nd edition. Edinburgh: W Green, 1999: para 8.53 where it is suggested that the jurisdiction in fact stems from the residual power of the Court of Session, the *nobile officium*. The *nobile officium* is a discretionary equitable jurisdiction exercisable by the Court of Session on petition to provide a remedy in civil actions where no remedy is available under existing law or statute. However, the judgments in Law Hospital NHS Trust v Lord Advocate 1996 SC 301 at 313, 1996 SLT 848 at 857E, [1996] 2 FLR 407, (1998) 39 BMLR 166, and in particular the statement of Lord Hope at 857E, suggest the power derives directly from the ancient power of the sovereign as *pater patriae* to protect the vulnerable.

60 Re F (Mental Patient: Sterilisation) [1990] 2 AC 1, [1989] 2 WLR 1025, [1989] 2 All ER 545, [1989] 2 FLR 376, HL.
61 Children (Scotland) Act 1995 s53(2)(b).
62 Children (Scotland) Act 1995 s54(2).
63 Children (Scotland) Act 1995t s52(2)(c).
64 Children (Scotland) Act 1995 s11.
65 Edwards L, Griffiths A. *Family law*. Edinburgh: W Green, 1997: 96.
66 Wilkinson AB, Norrie KMcK. *The law relating to parent and child in Scotland*, 2nd edition. Edinburgh: W Green, 1999: para 8.51.
67 While suggesting that courts should not be able to override competent young people's decisions, doubts have been expressed about how a court would resolve such issues. Sutherland EE. *Child and family law*. Edinburgh: T & T Clark, 1999: para 3.70; Thomson JM. *Family law in Scotland*, 3rd edition. Edinburgh: Butterworths/Law Society of Scotland, 1996: 168.
68 National Health Service in Scotland Management Executive. *A guide to consent to examination, investigation, treatment or operation*. Edinburgh: NHS in Scotland Management Executive, 1992: ch 2, para 14.
69 Scottish Law Commission. *Report on the legal capacity and responsibility of minors and pupils no 110*. Edinburgh: SLC, 1987: para 3.81.
70 Re F (Mental Patient: Sterilisation) [1990] 2 AC 1, [1989] 2 WLR 1025, [1989] 2 All ER 545, [1989] 2 FLR 376, HL.

4: Confidentiality

4.1 Patients' rights to confidentiality

All patients, regardless of their age, status or mental capacity, are entitled to expect that information about themselves provided or discovered in the course of their health care will not be revealed to others without their consent. Regarding the general duty of confidentiality owed to all patients, the General Medical Council (GMC) states:

> *Patients have a right to expect that information about them will be held in confidence by their doctors. Confidentiality is central to trust between doctors and patients. Without assurances about confidentiality, patients may be reluctant to give doctors the information they need in order to provide good care.*[1]

There is no simple legal basis for the duty of confidentiality, but the law is clear that the duties of health professionals in this respect apply to children as well as adults. As noted in chapters 2 and 3, the *Gillick* decision that it is lawful for doctors to give contraceptive advice and services to people under 16 confirmed that competent young people are entitled to confidentiality.[2] The law lords were in favour of parents being kept informed, but recognised circumstances where it would not be in the child's best interests for his or her parents to be told about a request for medical advice. Similarly the Human Rights Act 1998, which gives effect to rights in the European Convention on Human Rights (the "Convention rights"), forbids public authorities from interfering in a person's private life without legal authority or a legitimate aim. The Convention rights apply equally to children and adults. In Scotland, the Age of Legal Capacity (Scotland) Act 1991 is understood to imply that competent children are owed the same duty of confidentiality as adults (see chapter 3).

Children who lack the competence to give consent to treatment are also entitled to confidentiality. These patients should be encouraged to allow their parents to be involved but if they cannot be persuaded, doctors must judge whether disclosure to parents is necessary in the child's medical interests.

The GMC offers the following advice:

> *Problems may arise if you consider that a patient is incapable of giving consent to treatment or disclosure because of immaturity, illness, or mental incapacity. If such patients ask you not to disclose information to a third party, you should try to persuade them to allow an appropriate person to be involved in the consultation. If they refuse and you are convinced that it is essential, in their medical interests, you may disclose relevant information to an appropriate person or authority. In such cases you must tell the patient before disclosing any information, and, where appropriate, seek and carefully consider the views of an advocate or carer.*[3]

Research shows that worries about confidentiality dissuade some young people from approaching their doctor about health matters,[4] although this does not necessarily account for high teenage pregnancy rates since many teenagers who become pregnant have obtained contraceptive advice from their GP.[5] A consequence of concerns about confidentiality, however, can be that young people prefer to seek advice about sensitive matters such as contraception, sexually transmitted disease or drug addiction from specialist clinics, and do not allow those clinics to share relevant information with their GP. This can be detrimental both to the relationship between GP and patient and possibly also to the patient's health if, for example, the GP is aware of health issues that the patient does not pass on to the specialist clinic.

The BMA believes that teenagers' early uptake of sexual and other health advice and the liaison between services will improve if young people understand their rights and trust their general practice to uphold these. Practices should work to ensure that all patients understand that their health information will be kept confidential. Advice and suggestions for improving confidentiality in general practice, and for promoting the message to young people, are contained in a toolkit for general practice that has been produced by Brook Advisory Centres with the BMA, Royal College of General Practitioners and Royal College of Nursing.[6]

4.1.1 Deceased patients

The duty of confidentiality extends beyond a patient's death, although this does not mean that no information may be disclosed after a child has died. Information that patients asked to be kept confidential should generally not be revealed, but it is important that parents are able to find out the reasons for the death of a child. The GMC requires doctors to explain, to the best of their knowledge, the reasons for, and circumstances of, the death of a child under 16.[7] There is also a statutory right to copies of records relevant to a claim arising from a patient's death.[8] When considering disclosure after death, the likely impact of disclosure, or non-disclosure, on people who were close to the patient are important factors to consider.

4.1.2 Limits on confidentiality

The duty of confidentiality must be balanced against the interests of others and the wider community. Thus there are exceptional circumstances where information about any patient may have to be disclosed without permission. This need to balance the fundamental aims of preserving trust and preventing harm is reflected in all professional guidance. The exceptional cases where breach of confidentiality might be necessary can generally be described as disclosures "in the public interest", and include situations such as the prevention or detection of a serious crime, or the need to protect another person from a risk of serious harm. Confidentiality is too valuable a principle to be sacrificed for vague goals or indefinable harms, but where information can be used to protect people from serious harm, the principle may have to give way.

Whilst this concept of an exceptional and supervening public interest allowing some disclosures is widely acknowledged, nowhere is it closely defined. Outside the scope of obligatory disclosure, for example to comply with the law on notifiable diseases, each case must be considered on its merits. The BMA has produced detailed guidance on confidentiality and the disclosure of information, which offers further discussion of these matters.[9] In general, threats to people are significant in a way that threats to property or financial interests are not. Doctors must weigh the benefits and harms of disclosing information without consent, and must be prepared to justify any decision they make.

4.1.3 Involving parents

Notwithstanding wishes to keep some aspects of their lives private, most patients want people close to them to be involved in decisions about medical treatment. Ideally parents should help young people to make decisions about their health and should know when their child is receiving care. When children are young, parents, or parents and children together, make decisions. As children get older, they may wish to seek medical advice independently.

In all cases involving young people, health professionals should try to persuade them to allow their parents to be informed. Even when the young person is too immature to give consent to the treatment requested, the confidentiality of the consultation should still generally be maintained unless there is an overriding justification for not doing so. The medical duty of confidentiality is not dependent upon the competence of the patient and, unless there are very convincing reasons to the contrary, parents should only be told about their child's request for treatment, medication or advice with permission.

Parents clearly have rights to be informed to the degree necessary to fulfil their parental responsibilities, however, and the right to family life in the European Convention on Human Rights supports parental involvement in decision making (see chapter 2). In cases of conflict, the harms of breaching confidentiality must be weighed against the benefits of disclosure. For example it seems likely to be ethically justifiable to disclose information in order to allow a third party to give consent to essential treatment on the child's behalf. Nevertheless, a decision to disclose information against a young person's wishes is a significant one. Doctors may wish to discuss the issues with their professional, regulatory or indemnifying bodies.

4.2 Health records

4.2.1 Definition of health record

Health records are those records made by health professionals when caring for a patient, whether on paper, computer or stored in any other way. They include notes made during consultations, correspondence between health professionals such as referral and discharge letters, results of tests and their interpretation, x-rays, video tapes, photographs and other materials produced in the course of care. Doctors have obligations in respect of the information they hold, including the obligation to store and transmit it securely, and to provide access to it as appropriate.

4.2.2 Access to records

The law gives patients and, in some circumstances their proxies, the right to see and receive a copy of their health records.[10] The age of the patient is not relevant to rights of access and competent young people can exercise a statutory right of access to their own health records. Information must be withheld, however, in the rare circumstance that the health professional holding the record believes its disclosure is likely to cause serious damage to the physical or mental health of the patient or another person. Similarly no information that identifies or was given by a third party may be disclosed without the third party's consent, unless that person is a health professional who has been involved in the patient's care. Detailed advice on the statutory provisions is available from the BMA.[11]

Parental access

Any person with parental responsibility (see chapter 2 or 3) has a statutory right to apply for access to their child's health records. If the child is capable of giving consent, access may only be given with his or her consent. It may be necessary to discuss parental access alone with children if there is a suspicion that they are under pressure to agree. If a child lacks the competence to understand the nature of an application but access would be in his or her best interests, it may be granted. Parental access must not be given where it conflicts with the child's interests and any information that a child revealed in the expectation that it would not be disclosed should not be released.

CONFIDENTIALITY

There is no requirement to inform the other, perhaps absent, parent if access is sought, although if this would be in the child's best interests, it might be appropriate in some cases. General practitioners in particular can find themselves in a difficult position where separated parents, independently of each other, want information about their young child's health care. Some parents who do not live with their child ask the GP to contact them each time their child is brought to the surgery. There is no requirement on GPs to agree to such requests, which could entail a lot of time and resources if the child presents frequently. It is clearly better if parents are able to communicate with each other about their child's health, although doctors may agree to contact the absent parent under certain circumstances, for example if something serious arises. In any case, both parents may apply for access to the health records at reasonable intervals in time. Doctors are also usually prepared to discuss the child's health informally without requiring that the formalities of the legislation are followed. The aim is to ensure that both parents are involved in the child's health care without imposing a disproportionate burden on the doctor. Only if disclosure to either parent would be contrary to the child's interests should information be withheld.

A problem may arise if a young person who has been prescribed contraception refuses to allow her doctor to grant parental access to her medical record to conceal this fact, even though the doctor believes it would be in her best interests for her parents to be informed. Since the decision to prescribe in such cases turns on the competence and understanding of the patient, it would follow that a patient capable of making up her mind about contraception should also be able to control access to her health record. More difficult perhaps is the case of a young person who requested contraception that the doctor declined to prescribe on grounds of her lack of comprehension of what was involved. Such decisions are subject to the doctor's clinical judgment in each individual case, but unless there are very convincing reasons to the contrary, the doctor should keep this type of request secret even if the doctor believes the patient is insufficiently mature for the request to be complied with. If, however, the doctor considers the child to be at risk of exploitation or abuse, the limits of confidentiality should be discussed with her and information may exceptionally need to be disclosed (see section 4.3.1).

4.3 Circumstances in which confidentiality may need to be breached

The exceptional circumstances where it may be necessary to breach confidentiality arise where disclosing information will protect the patient or others from a risk of serious harm. Health professionals must weigh the advantages and disadvantages of disclosure versus non-disclosure and make a decision based on the individual circumstances. They must also be prepared to justify decisions, and be aware that they risk criticism for taking premature or inappropriate action as much as delaying taking action, where there are serious grounds for concern. If it is possible to do so safely, the need for disclosure should be discussed with the patient, who may be persuaded to disclose voluntarily. The situations in which information might be disclosed without the patient's knowledge are extremely rare. The BMA issues comprehensive guidance on confidentiality and disclosure of health information, which advises how to deal with situations such as disclosure to prevent serious crime, or preventing people from driving against medical advice.[12] These considerations are relevant to all patients. But specific issues arise in relation to vulnerable groups such as children and these are the focus of this section.

4.3.1 Confidentiality and suspected abuse

Abused children are entitled to have their confidentiality respected. A child or young person who comes to a doctor with a suspicious injury or other evidence of abuse should be the focus of the doctor's concern, not the family, although the doctor must also bear in mind the safety of others who might be at risk, for example the child's siblings. Some doctors say they feel a divided loyalty when they have as patients other members of the family, including the alleged abuser, but adults responsible for providing care have a duty to protect vulnerable people. Health professionals do not have statutory powers to intervene in family life, and so if intervention is necessary the matter must be passed to an agency that has the relevant statutory powers, namely social services or the police. Ideally this is done with the child's consent and cooperation.

Questions for health professionals where children are at risk of abuse or exploitation

- How can the child and others be protected from harm?
- Would further outside advice or intervention be helpful?

     If so, what is the best way of working with the child towards voluntary disclosure?

     If not, what support should the child be offered?

- Does the seriousness of the situation necessitate consideration of disclosure against the patient's wishes?

If health professionals are concerned about a child, they should provide support and counselling and encourage the child to agree, when ready, to information being passed to an appropriate agency. This task assumes greater urgency if the child, siblings or others are at risk. The child's rights to confidentiality should be explained, but it must also be emphasised that, where there are grounds for concern, there is a professional duty to take action to prevent serious harm to patients and others. Children and young people sometimes try to elicit a promise of confidentiality from adults to whom they disclose information about abuse. This is a common situation for health and other professionals who may be the first to be aware of a problem, but doctors cannot promise to keep information confidential if a child's safety is threatened. If time permits, discussion of the situation on an anonymous basis with colleagues and professional, regulatory or indemnifying bodies may be helpful.

If possible, the child should be given time to come to a considered decision about disclosure. If the child cannot be persuaded to agree to voluntary disclosure, and there is an immediate need to disclose information to an outside agency, he or she should be told what action is to be taken unless to do so would expose the child or others to an increased risk of serious harm. It is helpful if health professionals arrange a "safe" way to contact the child. Decisions about disclosure should be documented in the health records.

Where a child lacks the competence to make decisions about disclosure, doctors must protect that child's interests. It is clearly in the public interest to identify and prevent abuse of children. The GMC offers the following advice:

If you believe a patient to be a victim of neglect or physical, sexual or emotional abuse and that the patient cannot give or withhold consent to disclosure, you should give information promptly to an appropriate responsible person or statutory agency, where you believe that the disclosure is in the patient's best interests. You should usually inform the patient that you intend to disclose the information before doing so. Such circumstances may arise in relation to children, where concerns about possible abuse need to be shared with other agencies such as social services. Where appropriate you should inform those with parental responsibility about the disclosure. If, for any reason, you believe that disclosure of information is not in the best interests of an abused or neglected patient, you must still be prepared to justify your decision. [13]

Doctors should act in accordance with relevant guidelines and be aware, for example, of the work of area child protection committees. [14] The overall welfare of the child or young person must be the paramount consideration and his or her views must be heard but, as stated earlier, the child's own views are not necessarily the final arbiter in making decisions.

4.3.2 Child protection case conferences

The question of sharing information at child protection case conferences also raises dilemmas for doctors. The role of the doctor in such fora is seen as pivotal but frequently doctors are sceptical of the possibility of limiting the dissemination of information. Only information that is relevant to the purpose of the case conference and in the best interests of the child should be disclosed. Doctors will occasionally have to request that certain information is given in a limited forum or in writing to the chairman of the conference. Such measures should be used selectively for highly sensitive information and be avoided as regular practice.

Once matters have reached the situation of a case conference, parents and relevant carers are aware of the proceedings. Their cooperation over disclosure should be sought, especially if information about their physical or mental health is needed.

Examination and assessment for child protection purposes is the subject of appendix 1.

4.4 Use of health information for purposes other than health care

Care is needed where information about child patients is used for purposes not connected with their health care. If children object to their information being used, this should be respected. If information is used on the basis of parental consent, the child must be approached for permission for the information's continued use once he or she is competent to decide. A number of specific situations are considered below. Consent is also needed from parents if the information to be used, even indirectly, identifies them.

4.4.1 Teaching, audit and research

Consent for the use of personal health information in teaching,[15] audit or research should be sought from children who are competent to give it. It is usually inappropriate to use information about children if disclosure is contrary to their interests, or if the same objective could be achieved using information about adults. Where a child is unable to give consent, it must be obtained from a person with parental responsibility. If identifiable materials continue to be used over a period of time, the child's consent should be sought once he or she is competent to decide.

Involving children in research is discussed in chapter 9.

4.5 Visual and audio recordings

Recordings made as part of providing health care are subject to the same rules of consent and confidentiality as other medical treatment. The child, and his or her parents if they are involved, should understand that a recording is being made and what it will be used for. The GMC advises that there may be exceptional circumstances, such as where there is a strong suspicion of child abuse, where it may be in the child's best interests to make a recording without consent.[16] It may be helpful to discuss such situations with experienced colleagues, and doctors must be able to justify their decision to patients, families and others. At the time of writing, the Department of Health intends to issue guidance on the use of covert video surveillance, following a review of research practices at North Staffordshire Hospital NHS Trust.[17]

If recordings are made for purposes other than assessment or treatment, additional safeguards are necessary. The main principles may be summarised as follows.

Visual and audio recordings of children for purposes other than health care

- Doctors must be sure of the purposes for which videos or photos are taken and decide whether such purposes are valid.
- Valid consent must be obtained. Where children lack the competence to make decisions for themselves, parents should decide. If recordings are retained for future use, the child's consent for their retention and use must be sought when he or she has sufficient maturity and understanding. Refusals should be respected, and materials withdrawn from use if consent is refused.
- Consent should be sought for each and every purpose to which the recording is put.
- Where two-way screens are used either to monitor or film interviews, all individuals so monitored should be informed in advance and should know who is observing them and why.
- Recorded interviews should not be over-long and must be carefully managed.
- Ideally recordings should be made by registered medical illustrators, subject to a strict code of practice. Such people are usually aware of the potential legal and ethical difficulties involved and can help minimise the unease of the child or young person.[18]
- Recordings should be anonymised wherever possible.
- Identifiable material is confidential. It should be stored securely and used only for those purposes for which consent has been given.
- Competent patients should be aware of their rights in respect of the recording, specifically control over access and retention.

It is likely that parents and competent children may be able to exercise a statutory right to obtain a copy of recordings, if examination, diagnosis or treatment were involved. Further advice on access to information is available from the BMA.[19]

4.5.1 Media and publicity

Images of sick children may be used in the media for a whole range of purposes. Some are designed to benefit the child, such as in an appeal for donor tissue. Many images of sick children, however, do not aim to benefit the individual child but might be used to illustrate research findings, to promote information about a particular condition or unit, or purely for entertainment. Wherever possible, information should be presented in such a way as to conceal the identity of the individual patient, although consent should be sought for the use of even anonymous information where it relates to a specific individual (case studies, for example, as opposed to statistical or aggregated data).[20] From an ethical perspective, it is acceptable to use identifiable information about a child provided that the child's parents have given informed consent, the child agrees and it is not contrary to the child's interests either at the time or in the future.

Parents and children should both be involved in decisions about media contact. If a competent young person refuses to allow consent to be sought from his or her parents, publishers or journalists may be reluctant to proceed for fear of criticism from the parents after the material's use. Again, consideration must be given as to whether the use is likely to be harmful to the person's interests either at the time or in the future. Legal advice about proceeding without parental agreement is likely to be necessary.

4.6 Summary

Children and young people are entitled to the same standards of confidentiality as other patients. This means that their rights are not absolute but can only generally be overridden when there is a clear justification, such as the risk of significant harm. Where an exceptional reason justifies disclosure without consent, children should be told that their secrets cannot be kept. In the absence of any such reason justifying disclosure, they should be encouraged but not forced to share their health information with parents.

References

1 General Medical Council. *Confidentiality: protecting and providing information.* London: GMC, 2000: para 1.
2 Gillick v West Norfolk and Wisbech AHA [1986] AC 112, [1985] 3 WLR 830, [1985] 3 All ER 402, HL.
3 General Medical Council. *Confidentiality: protecting and providing information.* London: GMC, 2000: para 38.

4 Egg Research and Consultancy Ltd. *You think they won't tell anyone, well you HOPE they won't ... Do young people believe sex advice is confidential?* A report commissioned by Brook Advisory Centres and the Royal College of General Practitioners, funded by the Department of Health. London: Egg Research & Consultancy, 1999.

5 Churchill D, Allen J, Pringle M *et al.* Consultation patterns and provision of contraception in general practice before teenage pregnancy: case-control study. *BMJ* 2000;**321**:486—9.

6 To aim to improve young people's uptake of GP services the Department of Health funded a working party that met during 1998 and 1999 and produced materials to promote the message of confidentiality within the surgery, training materials for health professionals and other practice staff and suggestions for informing young people of their rights. British Medical Association, Brook Advisory Centres, Royal College of General Practitioners, Royal College of Nursing. *Confidentiality and young people. Improving teenagers' uptake of health advice. A toolkit for general practices.* London: Brook Advisory Centres, 2000.

7 General Medical Council. *Good medical practice.* London: GMC, 1998: para 18.

8 Detailed guidance on the provisions of access legislation is given in *Access to health records by patients.* London: BMA, 2000.

9 British Medical Association. *Confidentiality and disclosure of health information.* London: BMA, 1999.

10 Data Protection Act 1998.

11 British Medical Association. *Access to health records by patients.* London: BMA, 2000.

12 British Medical Association. *Confidentiality and disclosure of health information.* London: BMA, 1999.

13 General Medical Council. *Confidentiality: protecting and providing information.* London: GMC, 2000: para 39.

14 A number of specific guidelines have been published, including Department of Health, Home Office, Department for Education and Employment. *Working together to safeguard children.* London: The Stationery Office, 1999; Children's Legal Centre. *Child sexual abuse: a guide to the law.* Colchester: Children's Legal Centre, 1992.

15 The BMA issues guidance on the issues of confidentiality that arise when potential medical students observe medical practice. British Medical Association. *Work observation guidelines.* London: BMA, 1999.

16 General Medical Council. *Making and using visual and audio recordings of patients.* London: GMC, 1997.

17 NHS Executive, West Midlands. *Report of a review of the research framework in North Staffordshire Hospital NHS Trust* (Griffiths Inquiry). Birmingham: NHS Executive, 2000: recommendation, para 4.5.2.

18 The Institute of Medical Illustrators, a professional body for people involved in creating photographic and graphic images and audiovisual presentations within medicine and the health sciences, publishes a code of conduct. Institute of Medical Illustrators. *The code of professional conduct.* London: IMI, 1994.

19 British Medical Association. *Access to health records by patients.* London: BMA, 2000.

20 General Medical Council. *Confidentiality: protecting and providing information.* London: GMC, 2000: para 32.

5: Involving children and assessing a child's competence

We have emphasised that all children and young people who are capable of expressing preferences should be involved in decision making, whether or not they are the main decision makers. This raises questions, however, about the difficult task of trying to ascertain when a particular person is ready to accept information and make decisions affecting his or her life. In this chapter we look at ways of involving children and enhancing their ability to contribute to decision making, and also at the formal assessment of competence where doctors rely on a child or young person's consent to treatment.

The definition of competence is discussed in section 5.1. In general terms, people are competent to make decisions if they are able to understand the nature and purpose of the proposed treatment, and to retain the information and weigh it in the balance in order to arrive at a decision. In other words, whether a person is competent to do something depends on what that something is, and health professionals must look at the consequences and gravity of a decision when considering whether a person is able to make it.

Health professionals who assess ability to take valid decisions need to be skilled and experienced in interviewing young patients and eliciting their views without distortion. The treating doctor may be the most appropriate person, and other members of the health care team who have a close rapport with the patient have a valuable contribution to make. Any person whose opinion contributes to a formal assessment should understand the nature of the legal tests required. Where the courts are involved in competence and best interests decisions, it is usual to seek an additional opinion from a doctor acting as an expert witness rather than rely solely on the treating team's assessment.

The guidance given below is of a general nature and does not distinguish between hospital and general practice, nor between elective and emergency treatment. This means that not all of the factors listed are appropriate or relevant for every circumstance. It is not usually necessary to undertake a formal assessment of competence, but the ideas in this chapter for considering young patients' decision making abilities, and for encouraging them to be involved in decisions, are important in everyday practice.

5.1 Defining competence

As chapters 2 and 3 have shown, competence rather than age determines whether a person under 18 can give legally valid consent to medical treatment. All people over 16 are presumed to be competent to give consent[1] and those under this age may demonstrate their competence by meeting standards set by the courts.[2]

In England, Wales and Northern Ireland, a person under 16 is competent in law to give consent to medical treatment if the standard set in the *Gillick* case is met, in other words if he or she has sufficient understanding and intelligence to understand fully what is proposed.[3] In Scotland, statute says that a young person is competent if he or she is capable of understanding the nature and possible consequences of the procedure or treatment.[4] The High Court has also been clear that the test is whether the patient under 16 is capable of making a choice, not whether it is a wise choice.[5] The standard discussed in cases involving people over 16 is whether they are able to comprehend and retain information material to the decision, and able to use that information and weigh it in the balance as part of the decision making process.[6] In practice, all these tests are very similar. They turn on whether the patient understands the nature and purposes of the proposed treatment, and is able to weigh up the various factors relevant to the decision.

5.1.1 Coercion and undue influence

A competent decision must be free from undue external influences. Factors that might invalidate a choice include fear, confusion, shock, pain, fatigue, drugs, illness, medication, false assumptions and misinformation.[7][8] Influence is a particularly important consideration in assessing competence and health professionals should be aware that parents can exert great influence on their child's view of treatment. Health professionals themselves must try to avoid over-influencing children by providing biased or partial descriptions (see section 5.4.1). That is not to say, however, that decisions made with advice from parents or carers are necessarily in doubt. In the vast majority of cases people make decisions in consultation with people close to them and yet the final decision remains their own. What is important is whether the decision is the person's own independent choice.

5.1.2 The functional nature of competence

The definitions and the court's analysis of competence show that ability to take valid decisions depends on the decision in question. The nature and complexity of the decision or task, and the person's ability to understand, at the time the decision is made, the nature of the decision required and its implications, are all relevant. Thus the graver the impact of the decision, the commensurately greater the competence needed to make it.

5.2 A practical approach to assessing competence

General issues

- Competence is dependent on the task in hand. It should be constantly reassessed as children develop and as different treatments, tasks or challenges are faced.
- Doctors should be clear what test of competence is being applied and the nature of the task to be accomplished.
- Children of the same age differ significantly in their ability and willingness to participate. It is important not to approach young patients with preconceptions about ability.
- Consent, like treatment, is a process and not a single event, and doctors often have an ongoing relationship with a patient that allows for sound judgments about competence over time.
- Ability to participate can be enhanced by allowing time for discussion and ensuring that appropriate information is provided.
- Unless there are time constraints because of the nature of the illness, adequate time should be set aside so as to be able to explore the question of competence.
- Background information about the child or young person

that is relevant to the test should be obtained in advance, if possible. In particular, details about daily life and experience of illness may be helpful.

- Information from parents or carers who know and love the child or young person is of great importance, although doctors should be wary of relying solely on what could be an overly subjective view. Other people, for example teachers, play-specialists, nursing staff and social workers may be in a good position to provide an objective appraisal.
- Where GPs have known the patient for a long time, they may be well placed to evaluate competence and provide important information to other professionals about this. It must, however, be borne in mind that children constantly change and reliance should not necessarily be placed on an assessment that is not contemporaneous.
- A second opinion from a senior and experienced clinician may be helpful.

Assessment

Assessment of competence to take a specific decision regarding health care or treatment needs to be based on how that decision is dealt with rather than on any standardised tests (although these may be useful in alerting professionals to the possibility that a child is unusually mentally advanced or delayed in comparison with others of the same age).

Cognitive development

- The patient should demonstrate a concept of him or herself in relation to other people as shown by an ability to recognise, for example, his or her own needs and the needs of others. This might be shown by talking about relationships with parents, siblings, relatives and peers.
- The patient should recognise and understand that there is a choice to be made and show a willingness to make it.

Structured tests of cognitive development provide general information, although may not be task-specific.

Ability to balance risks and benefits of treatment

Some abilities develop as much by experience as by cognitive development. The assessment should consider whether the child or young person has:

- an understanding of what the illness means and that treatment is needed;
- an appreciation of what the proposed treatment involves and what the intended outcomes will be; and
- an understanding of the implications of both treatment and non-treatment and the consequences. This implies that the individual has a sense of him or herself over time.

These abilities might be demonstrated through talking about the illness, and about hopes and fears for the future. Assessors should be looking to see whether patients ask questions that show they understand, and/or whether they show understanding in response to direct questions from others. Play or drawings are a way for some children to reveal their level of understanding.

- Unwillingness to participate should not be interpreted as incompetence. A young patient who is competent to make his or her own decisions may nevertheless choose to allow parents to make decisions on his or her behalf. This demonstrates the ability to choose.
- Information must be retained for long enough to make an informed decision. This can be tested by asking questions about the information that has been given. A child may become irritated or bored by this, as might adults, but this is not evidence of incompetence.
- Some children are clearly unable to make decisions because of their immaturity or lack of ability to communicate their wishes. Extreme care is necessary, however, in making the assumption that the inability or unwillingness of a child to communicate with a doctor indicates incompetence.
- Doctors must be aware that their role as assessor can radically change the doctor–patient relationship and that if it is not handled sensitively there is a danger that assessment could undermine the trust, confidence and mutual respect on which the doctor–patient relationship should be founded.

The family

- Children and young people should be encouraged, and given opportunities, to discuss their health. This is particularly important for older children who may wish to discuss treatment without their parents.
- If cultural factors appear to be restricting the opportunity for

exchange between doctor and patient, for example if parents are unwilling to involve their child in decisions, doctors may have to explain why his or her involvement is important. Where families are not used to working in this way, this may require a great deal of time and sensitivity.

- Conflicts between people involved in the decision can hinder a young patient's ability to make a free choice. Discussion and attempts at achieving consensus can help.
- It is recommended that somebody other than a family member or friend is used where translation is necessary. If this is impossible, health professionals should be alert to the potential constraints that having a family member present might impose upon the young person's ability to speak freely.

5.3 Growth in level of understanding

Mental abilities, social understanding and emotional appreciation increase greatly during childhood development.[9] It is at about the age of two that children first develop a capacity to make inferences about the causes of events and to appreciate the psychological state of other people;[10] the ability to understand what other people are thinking increases markedly over the next few years.[11] Some commentators suggest that, from their first years, children think and feel deeply about their relationships and experiences and try to make sense of them,[12] and that children as young as five use understanding that adults rely on throughout life.[13] Strategic thinking and the ability to plan, however, do not become well established until later childhood or early adolescence.[14]

Anthropological research with children in many different societies illustrates how children's behaviours differ depending on the expectations and endorsement of their society.[15] Children and young people who are regarded as disadvantaged, such as those with chronic illness or disability, refugees and stigmatised or street children, may have opportunities to show their courage and maturity in ways that those growing up in a sheltered environment do not.[16] It is arguable that living in exceptionally challenging circumstances can reveal capacities that are latent in most children and young people.

Despite individual and even societal differences it is possible, and helpful, to make some broad generalisations about development. On the whole, younger children are more prone to be misled by leading questions and a wish to please adults.[17] The growth in mental abilities continues through the teenage years.[18] In early adolescence, young people are better able to think in an abstract, multidimensional, self-reflective and self-aware way and have a better understanding of relative concepts. This brings the ability to hold in mind several different dimensions of a topic at the same time, and so to generate more alternatives in decision making. In addition, as they develop, children become better able to monitor their own thinking for inconsistency, gaps in information and accuracy of logic. This greater mental sophistication that comes during the teenage years is accompanied by related developments in the ways in which young people think about themselves. During adolescence, there is a marked increase in emotional introspection, together with a growing tendency to look back with regret and to look ahead with apprehension. That is, not only do young people become increasingly able to consider the long term consequences of their own actions and of what happens to them, but also they tend to think about such consequences more in terms of their own sense of responsibility and to have a better awareness of the effects of what they do on other people.

These developments in intellectual capacities and emotions derive in part from continuing brain development (which extends well into the teenage years) and in part from life experiences. The increase in mental abilities reflects several different features, including knowledge base, ability to use more of the information available, more sophisticated mental planning capacities — which help in deciding how best to tackle decision making, and increased flexibility in the use of mental strategies.[19]

5.4 Factors affecting competence

Cognitive capacity and emotional understanding do not necessarily develop at the same rate. Also there is huge individual variation both in the time taken to reach particular mental levels and in the ultimate levels attained. Accordingly, no rule about competence that is based just on chronological age can possibly be satisfactory. This is true even for adult patients. The presumption of competence in people over 16 is rebuttable and decisions made by people who lack competence may not be determinative. The influence of emotional factors and experience on competence mean that mental age is not an answer either, although it may give better clues about competence than chronological age.

Standardised tests of understanding may underestimate what children and young people can and do achieve in more ordinary day-to-day situations.[20] This variation in mental performance is even more marked when the person's everyday experiences are unusual.[21] People tend to be very much better at solving problems when they concern issues familiar to them than when exactly the same problem is presented in an unfamiliar fashion. Also failure on a mental task does not necessarily mean that the relevant cognitive skill is missing. If children and young people can be helped to remember different facets of a decision making task, or if they can be shown how to adopt a different mental strategy, they may solve problems that are not ordinarily possible until a much older age.[22]

Much the same applies in the field of emotional understanding. Quite young children express mixed feelings but it is not until middle childhood that they gain much insight into their own emotional lives and realise when there is emotional ambivalence. Also, over the same age period, children learn a range of thinking techniques to control their emotions, although again, this is influenced by circumstances.

5.4.1 The role of information

We have said above that an important part of being able to make a decision is having the relevant information and being able to process that information. Giving and withholding information have been the subject of comment by the courts. In general, the courts have not criticised the deliberate withholding of information where it is believed that to provide it would cause extreme distress, as is shown by the case of L.[23]

Refusal of blood transfusion

In the case of *Re L*, a 14-year-old girl was severely burned by falling into a bath of scalding hot water, and refused the blood transfusion her doctors proposed. If she was not operated on, the medical evidence showed she would suffer gangrene and a slow and horrible death. L and her parents were Jehovah's Witnesses, and it was on religious grounds that L refused to accept the treatment. It appeared that the parents had not been asked to give their consent.

It was clear that L had not been appraised of the true consequences of refusing the proposed treatment. She was found by the High Court to lack competence with respect to this decision, and the transfusion was authorised.

Re L (Medical Treatment: Gillick Competence)

It is arguable that L, like A in the case of *Re E* discussed in section 2.3.2, was offered no real opportunity to consent. Information pertinent to their decisions about treatment was, albeit for compassionate reasons, withheld from them so they stood no realistic chance of being judged competent. These cases have been interpreted by some as professionals imposing incompetence on children by withholding the information necessary to make a competent choice.[24] Such action may be difficult to reconcile with the unlimited right to participate reflected in Article 12 of the UN Convention on the Rights of the Child (see chapter 1)[25] and rights under the Human Rights Act 1998 to receive and impart information (Article 10). These cases can also be interpreted, however, as the courts not insisting upon a full evaluation of competence where it might be contrary to the patient's best interests to carry out such an evaluation. In our view, information about health care should not usually be withheld from people who are willing to know it, although it may need to be provided gradually over a long period of time by somebody skilled in communicating with children. This allows the child or young person to adjust to specific issues before being told of the full gravity of a situation. Where, in exceptional cases, the harm of disclosure outweighs the value of seeking a competent decision, however, doctors may be justified in withholding relevant information.

In general, the choices patients make are strongly influenced by the manner in which the various options are presented to them and by the kinds of detail highlighted in those explanations. For all patients it is important that the information they are given about advantages and drawbacks of an intervention is accurate and balanced. Incomplete or very biased information may mean that patients cannot make a valid decision. Only where there is an overwhelming reason should information be withheld from patients who want to know it.

Essential information

As with patients of any age, how much information should be given to children and young people depends on the individual. Usually the following clear and simple explanations are relevant:

- an explanation or account of the condition/illness and its effects;
- a statement of the investigation or treatment that is proposed and its effects (which should include an explanation of the material risks and benefits, and chances of each occurring);
- an account of the risks and benefits of alternative, deferred or no treatment; and
- the practical consequences of treatment, including details such as the palatability of drugs, use of needles and blood tests, how pain will be relieved, effects on mobility, absences from school and effects on friends.

In some circumstances, parents, carers and health professionals may agree that it is not in a young patient's best interests to be told precise details of his or her diagnosis, although this is the exception, not the rule. A decision to withhold some information should not prevent the treating team from explaining in general terms the need for treatment and procedures and obtaining agreement for these. Children and young people need to feel that the treatment, however unpleasant, is better than the untreated illness.

5.5 Enhancing competence

Doctors are aware that competence can fluctuate and that there are many factors that influence the ability to make competent decisions. Barriers to competence and involvement can be overcome by providing the best opportunity for children to participate. The following suggestions and points may be helpful.

- Decisions may be easier if they are broken down into a series of smaller choices.
- Communication difficulties may result from physical disabilities, but can often be overcome. Careful assessment of speech, language functioning, hearing and sight can identify any potential barriers to communication. Translators should

be used where necessary, and should usually not be a member of the family, although in some cases this may be unavoidable. Independent translators can have an advocacy function, if appropriately trained.

- Written and other forms of recorded information can be helpful, and younger children may benefit from the use of play, drawings, games and puppets to help understanding.
- Children and young people differ, and may change their minds about the benefits of having a third party present in consultations and discussions. The competence of some young patients is enhanced by having a parent, carer or trusted member of staff present, but they should also be given opportunities to speak to the doctor or health care team alone.
- The venue should be non-threatening, welcoming and child-focused but not distracting. Anxiety about unfamiliar surroundings may mean that a child becomes frightened and less able to participate. Relatives or carers may have ideas about the most suitable venue.
- The doctor—patient relationship should be sympathetic, supportive and objective. An authoritarian relationship may inhibit young patients from expressing views.
- The way in which the child or young person is approached and dealt with generally can have a significant impact upon willingness to participate and capacity to do so. Health professionals are usually sensitive to this.
- Awareness of the family's usual pattern of decision making can be helpful; is it usual for the child or young person to play a significant part in decision making, and if not, how can he or she be encouraged and enabled to take on this role in the current situation?
- Vulnerability to coercive influences should be acknowledged and minimised.
- Competence and simply the ability to participate can be enhanced with treatment or symptom management. For example, management of pain or treatment of encephalopathy can mean a child is more able to take part. Similarly the effects of medication, for example euphoria induced by systemic corticosteroids, can affect competence. Whenever possible children and young people should be given the opportunity to express their views when any detrimental effects of medication are absent or at a minimum.
- Decisions should be delayed wherever possible and discussed

when a child or young person is best able to participate. Where competence fluctuates, children and young people should be consulted when they are at their most lucid and most able to participate.

- Depression and anxiety can be difficult to recognise, but may interfere with competence. Where there is doubt about mental state, a psychiatric opinion is often helpful.
- Competence is likely to improve over time, as the child matures and learns and understands more about health and treatment. Assessments of competence undertaken in the past are therefore unlikely to reflect current ability to participate.
- If a child or young person refuses to participate in health care decisions, efforts should be made to understand why this is the case and to overcome any difficulties or misapprehensions.

5.6 Summary

This chapter has set out some basic principles regarding competence, its assessment and involving young patients.

- Children and young people are competent to give consent to medical treatment if they are able to understand the nature and purpose of the proposed treatment, and to retain the information and weigh it in the balance to arrive at a decision.
- Competence is function specific. Doctors must therefore be aware of the task in hand when considering competence to make a decision.
- Whilst some children clearly lack competence due to immaturity, doctors should not judge the ability of a particular child on the basis of his or her age.
- Doctors should provide a child or young person with as much information about the illness and prognosis as is appropriate for that individual.
- Doctors should take steps to enhance ability to participate, and to encourage children and young people to do so.

In practice, formal assessment of competence as a discrete process is rare. Judgments about whether a young patient is competent to make a particular decision might be necessary if he or she presents for treatment alone, is to make the decision whether to accept or reject treatment options, or gives consent where parents refuse. The issue is less important in a legal sense if decision making involves the whole family and decisions are taken jointly.

The issues raised in this chapter, however, are about more than assessing competence. There are strong ethical and clinical obligations to encourage children to be involved in decisions about their health care to the extent that they are willing and able to do so. Using the techniques described here to enhance competence and facilitate participation are important aspects of good clinical care. Whilst these may appear to impose a considerable burden on the health care team in terms of being time- and labour-intensive, professionals should recognise that there is an increasing public demand for candour in health care. Educating, informing and involving children in health care decision making is an important investment with immense future potential benefits for the health service, its staff and its patients.

References

1 Family Law Reform Act 1969 s8(1). Age of Majority Act (NI) 1969 art 4(1). Age of Legal Capacity (Scotland) Act 1991 sl(1)(b).
2 Gillick v West Norfolk and Wisbech AHA [1986] AC 112, [1985] 3 WLR 830, [1985] 3 All ER 402, HL.
3 Ibid.
4 Age of Legal Capacity (Scotland) Act 1991 s2(4).
5 South Glamorgan CC v B, sub nom South Glamorgan CC v W and B [1993] FLR 574 , [1993] 1 FCR 626, [1993] Fam Law 398.
6 Re MB (Medical Treatment) [1997] 2 FLR 426, [1997] 2 FCR 541, [1997] 8 Med LR 217, CA.
7 Re T (Adult: Refusal of Treatment), sub nom Re T (Consent to Medical Treatment) (Adult Patient) [1993] Fam 95, [1992] 3 WLR 782, [1992] 4 All ER 649, CA.
8 Re MB (Medical Treatment) [1997] 2 FLR 426, [1997] 2 FCR 541, [1997] 8 Med LR 217, CA.
9 Ceci SJ, Bronfenbrenner U, Baker-Sennett JG. Cognition in and out of context: a tale of two paradigms. In: Rutter M, Hay D, eds. *Development through life: a handbook for clinicians*. Oxford: Blackwell Scientific, 1994: 239—59; Ceci SJ, Baker-Sennett JG, Bronfenbrenner U. Psychometric and everyday intelligence: synonyms, antonyms and anonyms. In: Rutter M, Hay D, eds. *Development through life: a handbook for clinicians*. Oxford: Blackwell Scientific, 1994: 260—83; Keating DP. Adolescent thinking. In: Feldman SS, Elliott GR, eds. *At the threshold: the developing adolescent*. Cambridge, MA: Harvard University Press, 1990: 54—89; Rutter M, Rutter M. *Developing minds: challenge and continuity across the lifespan*. Harmondsworth, Middx: Penguin, 1993; Walden T, Garber J. Emotional development. In: Rutter M, Hay D, eds. *Development through life: a handbook for clinicians*. Oxford: Blackwell Scientific, 1994: 403—55.
10 Kagan J. *The second year: the emergence of self-awareness*. Cambridge, MA: Harvard University Press, 1981.

11 Baron-Cohen S, Tager-Flusberg H, Cohen D. *Understanding other minds: perspectives from autism.* Oxford: Oxford University Press, 1993.

12 Bluebond-Langner M. *The private worlds of dying children.* Princeton: Princeton University Press, 1978; Alderson P. *Children's consent to surgery.* Buckingham: Open University Press, 1993.

13 Gardner H. *The unschooled mind.* London: Fontana, 1993.

14 Kail RV. *Memory development in children*, 3rd edition. San Francisco: Freeman, 1990.

15 James A, Prout A, eds. *Constructing and reconstructing childhood: contemporary issues of the sociological study of childhood.* London: Falmer Press, 1997.

16 Butler M. Negotiating place: the importance of children's realities. In: Steinberg S, Kincheloe S, eds. *Students as researchers. Creating classrooms that matter.* London: Falmer Press, 1998: 94—112.

17 Ceci SJ, Bruck M. Suggestibility of the child witness: a historical review and synthesis. *Psychological Bulletin* 1993;**113**:403—39.

18 Justice. *Children and homicide: appropriate procedures for juveniles in murder and manslaughter cases.* London: Justice, 1996.

19 Sternberg RJ, Powell JS. The development of intelligence. In: Flavell JH, Markman EM, eds. *Cognitive development, vol 3, Mussen's handbook of child psychology*, 4th edition. New York: Wiley, 1983: 341—419.

20 Dunn J. *The beginnings of social understanding.* Oxford: Blackwell, 1988.

21 Ceci SJ, Bronfenbrenner U, Baker-Sennett JG. Cognition in and out of context: a tale of two paradigms. In: Rutter M, Hay D, eds. *Development through life: a handbook for clinicians.* Oxford: Blackwell Scientific, 1994: 239—59.

22 Bryant PE. *Perception and understanding in young children.* London: Methuen, 1974; Goswami U. Analogical reasoning: what develops? A review of research and theory. *Child Development* 1991;**62**:1—22.

23 Re L (Medical Treatment: Gillick Competence) [1998] 2 FLR 810, [1999] 2 FCR 524.

24 McCafferty C. Won't consent? Can't consent! Refusal of medical treatment. *Family Law* 1999;**29**:335—6.

25 UN Convention on the Rights of the Child 1989 (20. xi. 1989; TS 44; Cm 1976).

6: Refusal of treatment and decisions not to treat

6.1 Refusal of treatment

Doctors propose treatment where there is evidence to suggest it might benefit a patient. Decisions about whether it should actually be given, however, may be finely balanced if the potential benefits are slim, or their degree uncertain. We have stressed in chapters 1, 2 and 3 that refusal of treatment by a child or young person who properly understands the implications is an important consideration to be taken very seriously, and that in Scotland that refusal may be binding on doctors. Where families support the child's decision this adds substantially to its weight, and such refusals are usually determinative if the implications of treatment are relatively insignificant for the child, either because the treatment is not essential or it offers only minimal or short-lived relief from a more serious condition. Refusal to participate in research or innovative treatment is discussed in chapter 9.

6.1.1 Refusal by parents

Decision making for children unable to decide for themselves is usually, and rightly, left to parents and the health care team. It is widely agreed that parents need time, respite facilities, possibly counselling, and certainly support from health professionals, but in most cases they are best placed to judge the child's interests and decide about serious treatment. Notwithstanding the importance of the parental role, however, where it appears that parents are following a course of action that is contrary to their child's interests, it may be necessary to seek a view from the courts. The courts recognise their duty to protect children and have almost invariably said that serious treatment should be given against the wishes of parents where there is a good chance of it succeeding (see sections 2.3.2 and 3.3.2). The courts are required, in their decision making, to have regard to the rights in the European Convention on Human Rights,[1] (the Convention rights) and to have the child's welfare as the paramount consideration.[2]

Consent allows treatment to be given, but does not require health professionals to treat. A decision whether to provide treatment on the basis of consent from one parent may be influenced by the view of the other. Although the law does not require that parents agree, in practice doctors are reluctant to override the strongly held views of a parent, particularly where the benefits and burdens of the treatment are finely balanced and it is not clear what is best for the child. Disputes between parents can be difficult for everybody involved in the child's care. Health professionals need to be able to distinguish between genuine concern of the dissenting parent and an objection that is simply an extension of a marital dispute. Discussion aimed at reaching consensus should be attempted. If this fails, a decision must be made by the clinician in charge whether to go ahead despite the disagreement. The onus is then on the parent who refuses treatment to take steps to stop it. If the dispute is over a controversial, elective procedure, for example male infant circumcision for religious purposes, doctors must not proceed without the authority of a court.[3]

6.1.2 Refusal by competent young people

Refusal of treatment by a child of any age should be taken very seriously and treated with respect, although it may be that in England, Wales and Northern Ireland the law will not uphold a competent minor's refusal of treatment.

Assessing the validity of refusal

- The patient must have both the information and the competence to make the particular decision in question.
- All the arguments should be aired and misperceptions or errors of fact discussed.
- The degree to which a refusal conflicts with the patient's welfare and overall best interests must be considered; some treatment refusal may coincide with a holistic view of best interests.

- Decision making should be open to question when it is seriously awry by the usual standards of what a reasonably prudent person in the patient's position would choose. Issues such as the young patient's desire to protect, please or punish other people should be addressed. Until there is evidence to the contrary, the presumption is that parents have their children's best interests at heart.
- Adults have a duty to intervene if children or young people appear to be exploited, abused and/or pressured by others. Emotional pressures on the child should also be addressed.
- A mechanism, such as referral to court, must exist for intervening in extreme cases if the young patient's decisions appear dangerous or seriously damaging.

If the expected outcome of a proposed procedure is relatively insignificant for the child in question it is unlikely to be justifiable to override his or her wishes. Where a competent young person refuses treatment, doctors should consider the impact of complying on his or her long term chances of survival, recovery or improvement. For example, an informed refusal of a procedure with a purely cosmetic outcome, or repeated chemotherapy that has not led to significant improvement in the past, is highly influential, whereas refusal of treatment that will substantially improve or prolong life is less likely to be the determining factor. Thus when deciding what is in young people's best interests where the likelihood of clinical success is uncertain, their informed refusal may tip the balance in favour of not giving the treatment.

It is difficult to envisage a situation in which it is ethically acceptable to provide elective treatment when a competent, informed young person consistently refuses it. There has been no guidance from the courts on this matter, as there has been no reported legal case dealing with refusal of elective or prophylactic intervention. This is likely to be because of the reluctance of doctors to impose non-essential treatment on reluctant competent patients.

Conversely, where non-treatment threatens life, or postponement would lead to serious and permanent injury, the ethical arguments for providing treatment against a young person's wishes are stronger. Doctors must act within the law and balance the harm caused by violating a young person's choice against the harm caused by failing to treat.

In UK jurisdictions where a young person's contemporaneous refusal of treatment may not be determinative, it follows that advance directives, or living wills, made by young people cannot be legally binding on health professionals. Young people may wish to express their wishes in advance, however, so that these can be given proper consideration in decision making and assessment of best interests.[4]

6.1.3 Refusal of blood products

Refusal of blood products is a sensitive issue about which health professionals express some uncertainty. Jehovah's Witnesses have a conscientiously held religious opposition to the use of blood products for themselves and their children but are generally very anxious to cooperate in every way with alternative options. Most Witnesses will not accept their own blood donated in advance (pre-deposit) but many are willing to accept the use of blood salvage equipment that serves to recycle their blood in a continuous circuit. "Bloodless" medical procedures are now becoming commonplace, including in recent years successful organ transplantations without blood.

The law

As discussed in section 2.3.2, the courts in England have overridden the refusal of blood by young people and their parents.[5] Lawyers in various jurisdictions, however, have drawn attention to the risk that health professionals may too rapidly assume that recourse to the courts to overrule a refusal — either by the child or by parents — is inevitably the only way forward.[6] This may mean that time is not given, even in non-urgent situations, to the exploration of potential alternatives to the use of blood. Jehovah's Witnesses also draw attention to what they consider to be an excess of caution on the part of health professionals that is manifested in too swift a resort to the use of blood when other alternatives may be available.[7] Health professionals should make every effort to accommodate beliefs rather than resorting to the most obvious medical option that is contrary to the patient's wish or looking to the courts as a first option. Nevertheless, where discussion, negotiation and consideration of other options fail to resolve the situation and a child's life is gravely at risk, it is likely that the courts will be involved. Courts have indicated that the administration of blood transfusions to Jehovah's Witness children against the wishes of their parents should not be carried out without the approval of a court.[8] Although these cases make no reference to the appropriate procedure in an emergency, Lord Templeman made the general point in the *Gillick* case that:

> *Where doctor and parent disagree, the court can decide and is not slow to act. I accept that if there is no time to obtain a decision from the court, a doctor may safely carry out treatment in an emergency if the doctor believes the treatment to be vital to the survival or health of an infant and notwithstanding the opposition of a parent or the impossibility of alerting the parent before the treatment is carried out.*[9]

Good practice

Clearly, wherever time allows, attempts should be made to negotiate with the family in an attempt to find an acceptable solution. Invariably, the family is anxious to save the child's life if this can be done in a way that does not contravene their beliefs. Sometimes, this may be possible by a referral to a specialist centre where techniques such as bloodless surgery are practised. Lists of current centres of excellence in such techniques and of doctors willing to work constructively with Jehovah's Witness families are held by the Jehovah's Witness hospital liaison committees. Hospital Information Services for Jehovah's Witnesses, a department of their coordinating body the Watch Tower Society, has published a summary of alternative therapies and references to the medical research that supports these.[10]

When faced with a refusal of blood products by or on behalf of a young patient:

- it is important that health professionals ensure that the situation is truly life-threatening and that there are no other feasible alternatives to the use of blood;
- the child and the parents should be given an opportunity to put forward their views and have these considered;
- the local hospital liaison committee for Jehovah's Witnesses, which may be able to advise on possible alternatives, should be contacted with the consent of the family or the competent young person; and

- if health professionals involved in the case consider blood products to be the only solution they can offer to save the life of the child, the patient or the patient's family may request that treatment be transferred to another facility where bloodless treatment is practised. Such wishes should be accommodated where possible.

As with all refusals of treatment, if patients are competent, informed and sure of their decision to refuse blood, there are significant ethical arguments for respecting this. The imperative to follow refusal by parents is necessarily weaker than when children themselves make informed decisions. Wherever time allows, there should be careful discussion with the young person and family to ensure that the situation is fully understood. Legal advice should be taken. It is advisable for health professionals to discuss the implications with the young person separately to ensure that a valid decision has been reached without any pressure.

6.1.4 Providing treatment when the patient refuses

As noted above, consent from somebody entitled to give it does not mean that treatment *must* be given. The harms associated with imposing treatment on a young person who refuses, whether competently or not, play a part in the decision about proceeding. How critical the treatment is, whether alternative less invasive treatments are available and whether it is possible to allow time for further discussion with the patient are all factors to be weighed. As much time as is practicable should be taken for discussion, and treatment delayed if that is possible without jeopardising its likely success.

If attempts to persuade a young person to cooperate with treatment fail, but it is judged to be in his or her best interests to proceed, it may only be possible to give the necessary treatment if restraint or detention are used. Such action may be lawful in certain circumstances but is rarely necessary. Even where there is resistance, talking to children and explaining why treatment is necessary usually helps them to come to accept, and cooperate with, the decision. Section 1.4.4 discusses the case of a 15-year-old girl, M, who refused to give consent for treatment and whose refusal was overridden by the court.[11] In authorising the doctors to proceed, the judge took great care to explain the reasoning in his judgment so M could see why her choice was not determinative. M later came to accept the treatment.

REFUSAL OF TREATMENT

Once a decision has been made that it is lawful and ethically acceptable to override a refusal of treatment, in principle there cannot be an absolute prohibition on the use of force to carry it out. However, "merely because treatment is in a competent patient's best interests does not mean the use of force is".[12] As has been noted throughout the book, the particular circumstances of a case and promoting the child's welfare in a broad sense are the overarching considerations.

Restricting liberty

Detention

A 16-year-old girl, C, who suffered from anorexia nervosa was the subject of a case in 1997.[13] She was receiving treatment at a private specialist clinic, but had a history of absconding. The clinic did not qualify as a hospital with powers of detention under the Mental Health Act 1983, and so sought an order from the High Court permitting the detention of C for the purposes of the provision of treatment. C was considered, by virtue of the nature of her condition, to lack the capacity to make decisions about her treatment.

The court held that C could be treated against her wishes and detained at the clinic for this purpose. Since she refused and was likely to attempt to abscond, the use of force to keep her at the clinic was authorised. It was acknowledged that detention was a "draconian remedy" and safeguards were required to ensure that force and restraint were the minimum necessary to achieve the aim, and that the period of detention should similarly be kept to a minimum. These safeguards were aimed at protecting C's welfare.

Re C (A Minor) (Detention for Medical Treatment)

Detaining children in a health care facility, outwith the provisions of mental health legislation (see chapter 7), raises legal issues because restricting the liberty of children is controlled by statute. A secure accommodation order may prevent certain categories of children from leaving a building or part of a building if a court determines that the criteria in the legislation are satisfied.[14] This applies to children who are looked after by a local authority (in care or being voluntarily accommodated) and certain others, including children accommodated by health authorities and NHS trusts.[15] Before making a secure accommodation order, the court must be satisfied that the child has a history of absconding and is likely to suffer significant harm if he or she does so again, or is likely to injure him or herself or another person. These provisions do not apply to children detained under mental health legislation, nor to certain children who are the subject of criminal proceedings. But otherwise, it is clear that court approval is necessary if a child is to be placed in a locked ward in a mental hospital, a regional secure unit, or other secure facility. A court asked to rule on such an issue is required to have regard to the young person's rights under the Human Rights Act 1998, and whether, in the circumstances, detention is compatible with these. A secure accommodation order does not authorise the child's treatment, and a separate legal justification must be found for any treatment.

The Department of Health issues guidance that acknowledges that there may be grey areas as to what constitutes a restriction of liberty.[16] It advises that any practice or measure that prevents a child from leaving a room or building of his or her own free will may be deemed by the court to constitute a restriction of liberty. One case that was taken to court, for example, concerned a 12-year-old child who was kept in an open adult ward in a nightdress, with her clothes locked in a cupboard.[17] While it is clear that locking children in a room or part of a building, to prevent them leaving voluntarily is caught by the statutory definition, other practices that place restrictions on freedom of mobility are not so clear cut. A variety of tactics that amount to restrictions on children's freedom of movement have been used in adolescent psychiatric units. In any case of doubt as to what constitutes acceptable restriction, legal advice should be sought and an application may need to be made to a court to determine the issue.

Using restraint or force

In addition to being difficult to achieve in practice, imposing treatment on young people where they refuse could damage the young person's current and future relationships with health care providers, and undermine trust in the medical profession. It is important for young people to understand that restraint of any form in order to provide treatment is only used as a matter of last resort, and not until other options for treatment have been explored. The child and the family must be offered continual support and information throughout the period of treatment.

Members of the health team benefit from being given an opportunity to express their views and to participate in decision making, although ultimate responsibility rests with the clinician in charge of care. All staff require support, and must not be asked to be involved in restraining a child without proper training.

If, after spending as much time as is practicable, it is impossible to persuade a child to cooperate with essential treatment, the clinician in charge of the patient's care may decide that restraint is appropriate. The following points are relevant to any action taken.

- Restraint should only be used where it is necessary to give essential treatment or to prevent a child from significantly injuring him or herself or others.
- Restraint is an act of care and control, not punishment.
- Unless life-prolonging or other crucial treatment is immediately necessary, the approval of a court should be sought where treatment involves restraint or detention to override the views of a competent young person, even if the law allows doctors to proceed on the basis of parental consent.
- All steps should be taken to anticipate the need for restraint and to prepare children, their families and staff.
- Wherever possible, the members of the health care team involved should have an established relationship with the child and should explain what is being done and why.
- Treatment plans should include safeguards to ensure that restraint is the minimum necessary to achieve the clinical aim, and that both the child and parents have been informed what will happen and why restraint is necessary.
- Restraint should usually only be used in the presence of other staff, who can act as assistants and witnesses.
- Any use of detention or restraint should be recorded in the medical records. These issues are an appropriate subject for clinical audit.

The Royal College of Nursing issues practical guidance on restraining children or preventing them from leaving that recommends that children and, where appropriate, parents and staff should be given the opportunity to discuss the incident as soon afterwards as possible.[18] The College also recommends that local policies on the use of containment and restraint should be developed.[19]

Restraint, if used in a prolonged or repeated way may amount to de facto detention, in which case, court approval is likely to be required (unless a child is formally detained under the Mental Health Act, see chapter 7). If restraint needs to be prolonged or repeated, urgent advice needs to be sought about the legality of effectively detaining a child contrary to his or her will. The Convention rights given effect by the Human Rights Act may have a bearing on how such an issue is decided.

6.2 Withdrawing and withholding treatment

The aim of medicine is to restore or maintain patients' health by maximising benefit and minimising harm. Treatment is offered if there is evidence of likely clinical benefit, although when treatment fails, or ceases, to provide a net benefit to the patient, this primary goal of medicine cannot be realised and the clinical justification for providing the treatment is gone. Unless some other justification can be demonstrated, most people would accept that treatment should not be prolonged, and that other alternatives, including palliative care and cessation of active treatment, should be considered.

6.2.1 Withdrawing and withholding life-prolonging medical treatment

Decisions to withdraw or withhold treatment are naturally most difficult where the treatment is likely to prolong life but it is not clear whether doing so benefits the patient. Advances in medicine continually extend the range of treatment options available to prolong life when organ and system failure would otherwise result in death. Cardiopulmonary resuscitation, renal dialysis and artificial ventilation prolong life and, for some children, allow time for natural recovery. For others, although with treatment they may remain stable for many years, there is no hope of the child ever experiencing more than a minimal level of awareness. Artificial nutrition and hydration are also forms of life-prolonging medical treatment, although many people perceive an important distinction between these and other treatments.[20] In recognition of how distressing and difficult these decisions are, and in order to reassure patients, their families and society that life-prolonging treatment is withdrawn or withheld in only those rare cases where provision would not provide a net benefit to the patient, decision making requires comprehensive safeguards.

The range of considerations relevant when assessing best interests is discussed in section 1.2. It includes the likelihood and degree of clinical success, the treatment's invasiveness and side effects and the wishes and needs of the family. Additionally some people believe that there is an intrinsic value in being alive and therefore that prolonging life always benefits patients, regardless of any other factors. The vast majority of children with even very severe physical or mental disabilities are able to, or may in the future, experience and gain pleasure from some aspects of their lives. Where it is clear that disability is so profound, however, that the child has no, or minimal, awareness of his or her own existence, no ability to interact with others, and no hope of achieving or recovering awareness, or where there is severe untreatable pain or other distress, it may be the case that prolonging life provides no overall benefit. The aim of the health care team then shifts to providing palliative care to ensure that the child has the best quality of life possible. How to identify the point at which the goal shifts in this way, and how to balance the benefits and burdens of treatment, are questions with clinical, ethical and legal dimensions. Decision making requires safeguards and review, and the aim of this section is to identify the relevant factors to take into account in decisions to withdraw or withhold treatment that has the potential to prolong life.

The BMA has published guidance on decisions to withhold or withdraw life-prolonging treatment: *Withholding and withdrawing life-prolonging medical treatment.*[21] Further advice has been issued drawing attention to the need to include consideration of the Human Rights Act in these and other decisions.[22] The advice that follows is a summary of those publications. The Royal College of Paediatrics and Child Health (RCPCH) also issues guidance on decisions to withdraw or withhold life-prolonging medical treatment.[23]

6.2.2 Clinical factors

Where treatment is unable to achieve its intended clinical goal, or imminent death is inevitable, active treatment provides no therapeutic benefit and may be withheld or withdrawn. The

RCPCH guidance identifies clinical situations in which it might be necessary to consider withdrawing or withholding treatment.[24] These include situations where:

- the patient is reliant on others for all care and does not react or relate to the outside world;
- treatment can only delay death with no significant alleviation of severe suffering;
- although the patient may survive, there is extensive physical or mental impairment that it is unreasonable to expect him or her to bear; or
- the burdens of further aggressive treatment for progressive and irreversible illness are believed by the patient and/or family to outweigh the clinical benefits.

All treatment decisions must be based on the best available clinical evidence. Factual information should be collected about the child's condition, diagnosis and prognosis, including the stability of the condition over time and the underlying pathology. Doctors must look to local and national guidelines on diagnosis and management, and on issues such as non-resuscitation decisions, to experienced colleagues if necessary, when assessing prognosis and considering treatment options.

Clinical assessment

Efforts should always be made to stabilise the child or young person's condition to allow for proper assessment and consideration of the likelihood and extent of any expected improvement. Where the evidence is clear that initiating treatment would be futile, this should be explained to children and their parents and future options for care and treatment discussed. Where there is reasonable doubt about the potential for benefit, treatment should be begun and the patient's condition reviewed. Openness with parents and carers about the purpose of initiating treatment where this is to assess its impact and effectiveness is important in case a subsequent decision to withdraw it is necessary.

Discussion of the possibility of having to face decisions about non-treatment should be routine at antenatal appointments so that parents and the health team are as ready as possible to make decisions in the labour ward should the need arise. As in all areas, decisions should be based on individual circumstances and the most recent evidence. Doctors should be wary of blanket policies that automatically deny active treatment to all babies below a given gestational age since these may be challenged under the Human Rights Act.

Having collected the necessary information, the type of factors that should be taken into account in the clinical assessment of benefit include:

- clinical judgment about the effectiveness of the proposed treatment;
- the likelihood of the child experiencing severe unmanageable pain or distress;
- the level of awareness the child has of his or her existence and surroundings and the likelihood of developing this;
- the likelihood and extent of any degree of improvement in the child's condition if treatment is provided; and
- whether the invasiveness of the treatment is justified in the circumstances.

Responsibility for decision making

Responsibility for the decision to withdraw or withhold treatment lies with the clinician in overall charge of the young patient's care. It is made in discussion with the family and the child or young person where feasible and appropriate. Where the decision relates to withholding or withdrawing artificial nutrition and hydration from a child or young person who is not imminently dying, there should also be formal clinical review of the decision by a senior clinician. The clinician should not be a part of the treating team, and should be somebody with experience of caring for children with the same condition. All decisions should be available for subsequent clinical review to ensure that appropriate procedures and guidelines were followed, and anonymous information should be available on request to the Secretary of State and, where applicable, the Commission for Health Improvement.

The same justification is required for continuing to treat as initiating treatment, namely that it provides an overall health benefit for the patient. Although emotionally it may be easier to withhold treatment than to withdraw treatment that has been started, there are no legal, or necessary morally relevant, differences, between the two actions. In other words, the emphasis in making treatment decisions should be on the reasons for providing it rather than on the justification for withholding or withdrawing it.

6.2.3 Ethical factors

The main decision makers in questions about withdrawing or withholding life-prolonging medical treatment are children, if they are able to participate, parents and the health team. Where the assessment of clinical factors does not provide a clear answer about whether the likely medical benefits of treatment outweigh its burdens, children and their parents are usually best placed and equipped to weigh the medical advice and apply it to their particular circumstances (see sections 2.3.2 and 3.3.2 for discussion of the limits on parental decision making).

Children's roles in decisions increase as their maturity and ability to express views develop. They should always be encouraged and helped to understand the treatment and care they are receiving and to participate in decision making to the extent to which they are willing and able. In almost every case, agreement about treatment is reached between the child, parents and the health care team. A lack of consensus can be a result of poor communication and inadequate provision of information to all those involved in the decision. Doctors should ensure that this is not the case. Additional clinical opinions, and discussion with other families who have experience of similar decisions can be helpful. Where serious disagreement remains after discussion, informal conflict resolution and additional advice, doctors are advised to seek legal advice about the requirement to obtain court approval before withholding or withdrawing life-prolonging medical treatment.

The traditionally accepted view is that nobody can ethically or legally insist on treatment that the health care team considers to be inappropriate or when the burdens of the treatment clearly outweigh the benefits for the child. In future it is possible that this will be challenged under the Human Rights Act. Whilst it is entirely understandable for parents to want to prolong their child's life for as long as possible, for desperate parents to expose fatally ill children to all manner of painful, unproven or essentially futile treatments breaches the child's right to be free from such intrusion. The doctor's first duty is to the child and in such cases the main task may involve gently helping the family to face reality.

6.2.4 Legal factors

Chapters 2 and 3 address in detail the legal matters of who can give consent to, or refuse, treatment on behalf of children and young people. Parents and young people are generally assumed to be the correct decision makers, although the courts may override decisions that seem contrary to the child's best interests.

The introduction of the Human Rights Act does not mean that life-prolonging medical treatment may never be withdrawn, but it does give legal force to rights that are relevant to decisions. The legitimacy of interfering with these rights is key in decision making, and doctors must be able to demonstrate that their actions are compatible with the Convention rights. In a legal case heard shortly before the Human Rights Act came into force, the courts considered whether a decision to withhold artificial ventilation from a baby was in breach of the Convention rights.[25]

Withholding of artificial ventilation

A baby, I, was delivered at 31 weeks' gestation by emergency Caesarean section for pre-eclampsia. He needed endotracheal intubation around 90 minutes after his birth, as a result of which he developed the well-recognised complication of ventilator-induced lung injury. Scans shortly after his birth also revealed irreversible brain structure abnormality.

He received regular mechanical ventilation during the first 50 days of his life, and then continued to need medical treatment, spending periods in paediatric intensive care. He suffered from severe, chronic, worsening lung disease, heart failure, hepatic disfunction and renal disfunction and severe developmental delay. When he was 19 months old, and in the face of serious and worsening disabilities, his doctors felt that further artificial ventilation was not in his best interests. It was clear that he would remain totally dependent for the rest of his short life. The doctors proposed that it would be best for I to receive palliative care to ease his suffering and permit his life to end peacefully and with dignity. His parents opposed this, and wanted I to be treated in a paediatric intensive care unit.

Referring back to previous cases in which non-treatment had been found to be in the best interests of the child, the High Court held that it would be lawful for artificial ventilation to be withheld if, in the opinion of the treating paediatrician, that was clinically appropriate.

A National Health Service Trust v D & Ors

Despite the Human Rights Act not having force at the time of the court's decision, the judge did look to the implications of the Convention rights on the situation, and concluded that his decision did not conflict with any Article of the European Convention on Human Rights. The judge explained that there could be no infringement of the right to life (Article 2) because withholding artificial ventilation was in I's best interests, and the right to be free from inhuman or degrading treatment (Article 3) included a right to dignity in death. The BMA anticipates that best practice in the withdrawing or withholding of treatment will not change radically following the Human Rights Act, which already requires benefits and burdens to be balanced, and the relevant parties to be consulted. Health professionals may be asked to justify their decisions on different grounds, however, having regard to the rights guaranteed by the Act. Information about legal developments is available from the BMA's medical ethics department and on the BMA website.

Persistent vegetative state (PVS)

Cases of children who are minimally conscious but in a stable state raise very particular difficulties in relation to balancing the benefits and burdens of treatment and the patient's Convention rights. Despite the voluminous medical literature and ethical and legal commentaries on PVS,[26] until recently very little guidance has specifically addressed the situation in relation to children. At the time of writing there have been no reported cases of applications to withdraw artificial nutrition and hydration from a patient clearly in PVS under the age of 18. Nevertheless, there has been considerable debate about general aspects of the condition in adults, including discussion about the value of rehabilitative efforts in the early phase before a diagnosis is finalised, and the importance of involving people close to the patient in decision making.

Guidance from the Royal College of Physicians notes that "it is a diagnosis which is not absolute but based on probabilities".[27] It states that the diagnosis "can be made at birth only in infants with anencephaly or hydranencephaly. For children with other severe malformations or acquired brain damage observation for at least six months is recommended until lack of awareness can be established". The RCPCH defines PVS as:

A state of unawareness of self and environment in which the patient breathes spontaneously, has a stable circulation and shows cycles of eye closure and eye opening which simulates sleep and waking, for a period of 12 months following a head injury or 6 months following other causes of brain damage.[28]

The RCPCH concludes that "treatment, inclusive of tube feeding may be withdrawn whilst making the patient comfortable by nursing care".

The English courts have indicated that, for the time being, all decisions to withdraw artificial nutrition and hydration from patients in PVS or a state of very low awareness closely resembling PVS should come before the courts. This is an interim measure until a body of experience in dealing with the condition has developed, and until other effective mechanisms for decision making are in place. The courts in Scotland have not made court review a formal requirement, although this is desirable for cases involving children and young people. Although ideally reliance on widely accepted professional guidance, and robust mechanisms for decision making and review are preferable to involving the courts, uncertainty about the condition in children means that court review provides a welcome safeguard for those who have to face these difficult decisions. Legal advice is essential.

Do not resuscitate orders

Another area of decision making that deserves separate mention is cardiopulmonary resuscitation (CPR) and do-not-resuscitate (DNR) orders. The BMA advises health care facilities to establish local policies to cover the involvement of patients and families in decisions. Such policies should also clarify situations in which consideration of a DNR order is appropriate, responsibility for decision making and communication of the decision to families and the health care team.[29] All guidelines must also cover the impact of the Human Rights Act and how this highlights the need for transparency and openness.

6.2.5 Once a decision has been made

If agreement is reached that ceasing further active or invasive treatment is best for a child or young person, all those involved in the decision, the patient, parents, other relatives and the health care team, should be informed of the decision and its basis. This explanation can help those involved in caring for the child to satisfy themselves that the decision is right. It can also help people close to the child come to terms with the situation. Discussion gives advance notice of any disagreement about the decision and provides an opportunity to identify whether there is a need for further clinical advice or legal review.

It is essential to emphasise that the decision does not represent abandoning or "giving up on" the child but rather that other forms of care are more appropriate. It is the value of the treatment that is being assessed, not the value of the child. Although the immediate goal may, rightly, have shifted from seeking the benefits that arise from prolonging life to seeking those that arise from being comfortable and free from pain, the overall objective of providing benefit does not change.

A decision to withdraw or withhold treatment is not immutable, although its effects once implemented may be irreversible. The situation must be reviewed both before and after implementation to look for and take account of any change in circumstances. The decision, its basis and subsequent change must be recorded in the medical record. Decisions to withdraw or withhold treatment are an appropriate subject for clinical audit.

Where a member of the health care team has a conscientious objection to the proposed course of action, that person should, wherever possible, be permitted to hand over his or her role in the care of the child to a colleague. Health professionals involved in the decision, as well as family members, can be left with feelings of guilt and anxiety as well as bereavement, and it is important there is support available both before and after the decision to withdraw or withhold treatment has been made. It is essential that bereavement counselling is available for families.

6.3 Summary

6.3.1 Refusal of treatment

Decisions about whether treatment should be offered to a child and his or her family are commonplace. It is part of routine medical care to assess the benefits a treatment is offering and to balance these with the needs and wishes of children and their families. The decisions become particularly difficult where the benefits and burdens are finely balanced, for example where there is only a slim chance that a particularly invasive treatment will result in, even limited, improvement in a serious condition, or when agreement about how to proceed cannot be reached. The aim of decision making is always to reach consensus. In the rare cases where this cannot be achieved despite all efforts, the courts may intervene.

- All efforts should be made to overcome disagreements about treatment.
- Refusal by a child or parent is an important factor in the assessment of best interests.
- The harm caused by violating a competent choice must be balanced against the harm caused by failing to treat.
- It is unlikely to be ethically justifiable to override a young person's sustained, competent and informed refusal of treatment unless the treatment is essential to save or significantly enhance life.
- Providing treatment to a competent young person against his or her wishes may require the approval of a court, particularly if providing it requires the use of restraint or restriction of liberty.

6.3.2 Withdrawing and withholding treatment

- There is no obligation on health professionals to offer medical treatment that cannot achieve its clinical aim, or that cannot provide an overall benefit to the child.
- In deciding whether treatment should be begun or stopped, health professionals must act within the law and take the lead in assessing the relevant clinical factors.
- Decisions about best interests more broadly are made by families, with the influence of the views of young people growing with their maturity and understanding of the decision.
- Support for the child, the family and health care team is essential throughout the process of deciding about the provision of life-prolonging treatment, and during and following its implementation.
- In making such decisions, consideration must be given to the Human Rights Act.

Whether the reason for not giving active treatment is because it can provide no clinical benefit to the child, or because the child, the parents and the health team agree it is not in the child's best interests, children must never be abandoned. Other treatment and care options should be discussed, and palliative care must be available for all children who are dying.

References

1 Convention for the Protection of Human Rights and Fundamental Freedoms (4. ix. 1950; TS 71; Cmnd 8969).

2 Children Act 1989 s1(1). The Children (Northern Ireland) Order 1995 art 3(1). Children (Scotland) Act 1995 s16(1).

3 Re J (A Minor) (Prohibited Steps Order: Circumcision), sub nom Re J (Child's Religious Upbringing and Circumcision) and Re J (Specific Issue Orders: Muslim Upbringing & Circumcision) [2000] 1 FLR 571; [2000] 1 FCR 307; (2000) 52 BMLR 82. The BMA issues guidance for doctors on male infant circumcision that is available on request and on the BMA website, www.bma.org.uk.

4 The BMA publishes general guidance on advance decision making in: British Medical Association. *Advance statements about medical treatment.* London: BMA, 1995.

5 Additional cases not referenced in the earlier chapters include: Re O (A Minor) (Medical Treatment) [1993] 2 FLR 149, [1993] 1 FCR 925, [1993] 4 Med LR 272; Re S (A Minor) (Medical Treatment) [1993] 1 FLR 377, [1993] Fam Law 215; Re R (A Minor) (Blood Transfusion) [1993] 2 FLR 757.

6 See for example, Pansier F-J. The legal relationship of the patient and physician in bloodless surgery. In: Pansier F J. *Bloodless surgery: surgical and anaesthetic aspects, legal and ethical issues.* Paris: Arnette Blackwell SA, 1997.

7 Watch Tower Bible and Tract Society of Pennsylvania. *Family care and medical management for Jehovah's Witnesses.* New York: Watch Tower Bible and Tract Society of New York, 1995.

8 Re O (A Minor) (Medical Treatment) [1993] 2 FLR 149, [1993] 1 FCR 925, [1993] 4 Med LR 272; Re S (A Minor) (Medical Treatment) [1993] 1 FLR 377, [1993] Fam Law 215.

9 Gillick v West Norfolk and Wisbech AHA [1986] AC 112 at 200G; [1985] 3 WLR 830; [1985] 3 All ER 402, HL.

10 Watch Tower Bible and Tract Society of Pennsylvania. *Family care and medical management for Jehovah's Witnesses.* New York: Watch Tower Bible and Tract Society of New York, 1995.

11 Re M (Child: Refusal of Medical Treatment) [1999] 2 FLR 1097, [1999] 2 FCR 577.

12 Grubb A. Commentary: court's inherent jurisdiction (child): detention and treatment, *Medical Law Review* 1997;5:227—33.

13 Re C (A Minor) (Medical Treatment: Court's Jurisdiction), sub nom Re C (A Minor) (Detention for Medical Treatment) [1997] 2 FLR 180, [1997] 3 FCR 49, [1997] Fam Law 474. The issues of force were also addressed in Wolverhampton MBC v DB (A Minor), sub nom Re B (A Minor) (Treatment and Secure Accommodation), A MBC v DB [1997] 1 FLR 767, [1997] 1 FCR 618; (1997) 37 BMLR 172. In that case, the court authorised the use of force to treat a 17-year-old drug addict who required a Caesarean section and other medical treatment to preserve her life and health.

14 Children Act 1989 s25. The Children (Northern Ireland) Order 1995 art 44. Children (Scotland) Act 1995 s57 and 70. For explanation, see, for example, Department of Health. *The Children Act 1989 guidance and regulations. Volume 4. Residential care.* London: HMSO, 1991: para 8.10. R v Northampton Juvenile

Court ex parte London Borough of Hammersmith and Fulham [1985] FLR 193, [1985] 1 Fam Law 124.

15 Children Act 1989 s25(7)(a). Children (Secure Accommodation) Regulations 1991 (SI 1991/1505) Regulation 7(1)(a). The health authority or NHS trust providing the accommodation must make the application to court. Children (Secure Accommodation) (No. 2) Regulations 1991 (SI 1991/2034). The Children (Northern Ireland) Order 1995 art 44(8)(a). Children (Secure Accommodation) Regulations (NI) 1996 (SR 1996/487). Children (Scotland) Act 1995 s57 and 70.

16 Department of Health. *The Children Act 1989 guidance and regulations. Volume 4. Residential care*. London: HMSO, 1991: para 8.10.

17 R v Kirklees MBC ex parte C [1993] 2 FLR 187, [1993] 2 FCR 381, [1993] Fam Law 453.

18 The Royal College of Nursing. *Restraining, holding still and containing children: guidance for good practice*. London: RCN, 1999.

19 An example of such a policy has been developed by a working party in the Southampton and South West Health District. Southampton Community Health Service Trust & Hampshire County Council Social Services. *Children and adolescents and mental health practice handbook*. 1996.

20 Artificial in this context means ways of providing nutrition and hydration that bypass the swallowing mechanism, for example nasogastric tubes, percutaneous endoscopic gastrostomy (PEG feeding) and total parenteral nutrition. Oral nutrition and hydration, on the other hand, where food or nutritional supplements are offered into the patient's mouth, is an aspect of basic care. This and other aspects of basic care must never be withdrawn.

21 British Medical Association. *Withholding and withdrawing life-prolonging medical treatment*, 2nd edition. London: BMJ Books, 2000. The full text of this publication can be found at www.bmjpg.com/withwith/ww.htm.

22 British Medical Association. *The impact of the Human Rights Act on medical decision making*. London: BMA, 2000.

23 Royal College of Paediatrics and Child Health. *Withholding or withdrawing life saving treatment in children: a framework for practice*. London: RCPCH, 1997.

24 Ibid.

25 A National Health Service Trust v D & Ors (2000) TLR 19 July 2000.

26 See for example, Walsh P. *The vegetative state: persisting problems in law and regulation*. London: King's College, 1999, which summarises European guidelines on this issue as well as recent American literature.

27 Royal College of Physicians. The permanent vegetative state. *Journal of the Royal College of Physicians* 1996;30:119–21. This article also reflects disagreement about terminology. Some organisations, including the BMA continue to refer to the "persistent" vegetative state. The Royal College of Physicians uses "permanent" and some legal commentators simply refer to "the vegetative state".

28 Royal College of Paediatrics and Child Health. *Withholding or withdrawing life saving treatment in children: a framework for practice*. London: RCPCH, 1997: 7.

29 British Medical Association, Resuscitation Council (UK), Royal College of Nursing. *Decisions relating to cardiopulmonary resuscitation*. London: BMA, 1999.

7: Mental health care of children and young people

The focus in this chapter is primarily on ethical and practical issues that arise for health professionals providing assessment and mental health care for children and young people. We follow the convention of other reports[1] and use the term "mental health problem" generically to cover a range of types and severity of psychological and psychiatric disorders in children and young people. Clearly, the widely different types of disorder subsumed under this heading preclude us from mentioning specific treatment options in anything more than a very generalised manner. Management of emotional disorders, such as phobias, is clearly very different from the management of conduct disorders or development disorders, such as autism, or psychotic disorders, such as schizophrenia. Therefore, this chapter is limited to a summary of some general principles, interspersed with some illustrative case histories. We begin by considering general good practice in this sphere of care before considering the problematic decisions that arise and potential solutions. Some aspects of law are mentioned in this chapter and it should be noted that the law in Scotland differs from that in England, Wales and Northern Ireland. (The relevant equivalent legislation in Scotland to the statutes mentioned in this chapter are the Children (Scotland) Act 1995, the Mental Health (Scotland) Act 1984, the Age of Legal Capacity (Scotland) Act 1991 and the Adults with Incapacity (Scotland) Act 2000. For clarity, this chapter refers to the English legislation, but highlights that of other UK jurisdictions where matters of principle differ.) A general discussion of the law and the principal differences between Scotland and the rest of the UK can be found in chapters 2 and 3.

7.1 Good practice

7.1.1 The relevance of general ethical principles

It is important to emphasise that the same basic ethical principles governing the medical care of children and young people apply in mental health care as elsewhere. The principles also apply equally to patients with mental illness and learning disability. They include the necessity of providing information to young patients, in an accessible way, and listening to their views. Wherever possible, the use of compulsory powers contrary to the patient's wishes should be avoided and, where feasible, health professionals should try to comply with patients' wishes or negotiate with them to find an acceptable compromise. As in other spheres of treatment, the establishment of a collaborative, trusting relationship with the patient is a priority. Therefore, wherever it is feasible to do so, the young person should be involved in the discussion even though he or she will not necessarily have the casting vote about what happens. Families should be involved in therapy decisions, wherever possible. Also, as with all other treatments, if a young person is judged to lack the competence to make a valid decision about a particular issue, a solution is sought based on an assessment of the patient's best interests (see chapter 1).

As in all other spheres of treatment, health professionals have an obligation to encourage patients to be involved in weighing up the options and using to the full their own decision making capacity. The fact that a patient is considered not able to make a valid decision about one aspect of care or treatment does not imply that the same person cannot make other perfectly valid treatment decisions. Just as with other areas of care, treatment in this sphere should be the least invasive possible, the least restrictive of the individual's freedom and should be based on evidence of efficacy. Treatment regimes should aim to separate the child as little as possible from family, friends, school and community contacts. Some of these principles are particularly emphasised in the Mental Health Act Code of Practice and are applicable to young patients with a mental illness or a learning disability.[2]

Guiding principles in the Mental Health Act code of practice

- Children should be fully informed about their care. Their

views should be sought and taken into account. The impact of the child's wishes on parents (or other people with parental responsibility) should always be considered.

- Any intervention should be the least restrictive possible and should segregate the child as little as possible from family, friends, community and school.
- All children in hospital should receive appropriate education.

In addition, established good practice should also reflect the following points.

Good practice should be based on:

- evidence of efficacy;
- equitable access;
- service acceptability to enable optimal patient compliance with treatment;
- maintenance of staff skills and morale;
- planned and agreed prioritisation of cases;
- holistic management of the child and awareness of relevant contextual factors;
- maximum participation of the child in decisions with full consideration being given to the child's wishes; and
- optimal use of resources.

7.1.2 Establishing trust

Young patients should be involved as much as possible in the planning of their own care and treatment regimes, in conjunction with their families. Clearly, the needs of each patient must be assessed on an individual basis and the approach to treatment must reflect those specific needs.

Nevertheless, mutual trust can be hard to establish with patients who have a completely different view of reality from that of the health professionals treating them. Patients with eating disorders, for example, suffer from a condition that not only affects how they see themselves but impinges on their behaviour in a way that can result in death. They may exhibit a level of general understanding that is more than adequate to grasp the issues but still be hampered in regard to compliance with treatment regimes because of their own distorted perceptions. Throughout this book, attention has been drawn to the importance of fully evaluating the patient's competence to make a valid choice. In some cases, however, although patients may understand the treatment and the consequences of failure to accept it, the effects of their illness undermine their ability to make an informed choice. A needle phobia, for example, can prevent the patient from accepting essential treatment while understanding the need for it. As Lady Justice Butler-Sloss has pointed out, "panic induced by fear" can undermine an otherwise competent patient's ability to accept treatment since fear may "paralyse the will and destroy the capacity to make a decision".[3] Anorexia nervosa can create in the sufferer a compulsion to refuse treatment or only to accept treatment that is likely to be ineffective. In cases of anorexia, poor nutrition can result in cognitive impairment that further impinges on the child's ability to make rational decisions.[4] Among the ethical and practical dilemmas facing health professionals treating this group of patients is when to judge that the collaborative approach can no longer be sustained. Clearly, the objective is always to maintain a relationship based on patient consent and negotiation, even though this may entail allowing the patient to take some health risks. At some point, however, the risks become untenable and health professionals have to take over responsibility.

Case example

X was a competent and articulate young woman suffering from an eating disorder. The option of inpatient treatment was discussed with X and her family, who were all in agreement that it was essential to her long term health. Nevertheless, X wished to postpone admission to the unit until she had reached a particular low weight goal. She felt that if she were able to achieve this low weight, even temporarily, it would enable her to overcome her weight obsession and put it behind her. The health team and X's family agreed to allow her to try this option as long as she agreed to cooperate with treatment as soon as she reached that weight or sooner if her health seemed jeopardised. Initially, therefore, the health team were in the paradoxical position of supporting X in her attempt to lose more weight. Before she reached her goal, X became increasingly ill and after discussion agreed to be admitted for inpatient care once she had reached a compromise weight that was higher than her original goal. Although the health team discussed the various options for overruling

---

X's efforts to postpone treatment, including use of the Mental Health Act, it was agreed that until the health risks for X became too great they would attempt to maintain supervision and treatment on a voluntary basis, even though this required frequent renegotiation.

(Unreported case)

7.2 The patient population under consideration

The number of children suffering from mental health problems is estimated to be considerable as has been indicated by various studies over the past 20 years. Nevertheless, it remains difficult to obtain a full picture of the extent of such problems within the childhood population at any time. Some studies have focused on the likely extent of the problem in a particular age group of children while others looked at numbers of children with a particular form of mental disorder. In order to be useful, statistics concerning prevalence need to take account of variations according to clinical and social risk factors such as genetics, brain injury, abuse, bereavement and homelessness. Clearly, such risks vary according to a number of factors, including geographical and social situation. For example, consistently higher rates of childhood mental health problems have been found in urban, as opposed to rural, areas. A national psycho-morbidity study published by the Office for National Statistics (ONS) in 2000, suggested that around 10 percent of 5—15 year olds in England, Scotland and Wales experience some type of mental disorder.[5] Even this study, however, does not give the whole picture as experts in this area, Harbour and Bailey, point out.[6] While the ONS study looked at the prevalence of a specific group of disorders, it excluded the types of mental disorder that commonly justify detention under the Mental Health Act, such as early onset psychosis.

7.2.1 Risk of social stigma

Health professionals are very aware of the potential stigma attached to a diagnosis of mental illness. Attention is often drawn to the "reluctance to diagnose psychiatric disorder owing to fears about the adverse effects of medical labelling and stigmatisation".[7] There is still hesitation about invoking the Mental Health Act for children and young people. Most objections focus on the potentially stigmatising effect. While this cannot be dismissed as a risk, it must be balanced against the benefits accorded to patients by the statutory safeguards in the Act.

Early and accurate diagnosis is essential for early intervention, which in turn is crucial for successful treatment. It can be argued that it is the fact of having a "mental disorder" recorded in a patient's notes, or the perception that an individual may be predisposed to dangerous behaviour, that are potentially stigmatising, rather than the use of the Mental Health Act. The issue of stigma should be carefully considered by the health care team in consultation with parents, and the child, if practicable.

7.2.2 Confidentiality

Because of the potentially stigmatising effect of treatment for a mental disorder, patient confidentiality is particularly important in this area but it is also an area of practice where confidentiality seems hard to protect. Some of the practical difficulties arise because some forms of therapy involving competent young people are family-based and designed to include family therapy or parental counselling. Treatment may involve encouraging patients to air with their parents important issues that they are exploring with their key workers. Obviously, patients need to be able to do this at their own pace.

The Mental Health Act Code of Practice emphasises that "children's rights to confidentiality should be strictly observed. It is important that all professionals have a clear understanding of their obligations of confidentiality to children and that any limits to such an obligation are made clear to a child who has the capacity to understand them".[8] Exceptional circumstances may arise where it becomes necessary to disclose information without consent, to protect either the patient or other people from serious harm. Disclosure in such situations should follow the same principles as non-consensual disclosure in all other circumstances and where possible, the patient should be informed in advance of the need to breach confidentiality and why (see chapter 4). Generally speaking, confidentiality should only be breached contrary to the patient's wishes when issues of safety arise. Nevertheless, as in all other areas of care, good liaison and communication between different agencies is essential. A range of professionals may need to be kept informed following the child's discharge from inpatient care, including the GP, the local psychiatric service, social services and schools. Patients may be particularly sensitive about how information concerning their mental health is used and more anxious about this than they would be were their illness purely physical. Therefore, they need to have a say in how information will be shared.

7.3 Consent and refusal of mental health care

As made clear at the beginning of the chapter, the provision of information in order to facilitate valid consent is as important in this sphere of care as in others. Clearly, special care is needed when attempting to involve children with learning disabilities or those whose reasoning skills may be affected by illness. Health professionals have an obligation to make all reasonable efforts to enhance patients' competence and to encourage them to use to the full the decision making abilities they possess (see section 5.5). An expert committee set up by the government to review the mental health legislation in England and Wales made a series of recommendations in 1999 in relation to the mental health care of children and young people.[9] Among these recommendations was the concept of a rebuttable presumption of capacity in children from the age of 10 or 12 to make treatment decisions. If adopted, this would mean that from that age, children would be presumed to have sufficient competence to decide on questions of medical treatment, unless the contrary could be shown to be true in the case of a particular child. At present, the presumption of competence arises at age 16 (see sections 2.2 and 3.2).

Treatment of a child who lacks competence: As with other treatments, a child who is not capable of making his or her own decisions can usually be treated with the consent of a parent, or another person with parental responsibility. If the person with parental responsibility cannot be found or if that person is not acting in the child's interests or also lacks competence, the courts may need to be involved.

Consent by a competent child: The ideal treatment plan involves the voluntary consent of the child or young person. The fact that a patient suffers from a mental disorder does not necessarily mean that he or she cannot give valid consent to treatment. Consent should always be sought when the patient is treated under the Mental Health Act. Use of statutory powers does not preclude the implementation of the principles of good practice. When patients properly understand the reason for treatment and the risks of non-compliance, they are more likely to cooperate with the treatment regime. Sensitivity, honesty and trust between doctor and patient are vital to effective cooperation.

Refusal by a competent child: In some cases, it may be possible to negotiate an acceptable treatment compromise when a competent child refuses the proposed option. In England, Wales and Northern Ireland, children or young people under 18 cannot normally override a consent to treatment given on their behalf by anyone who has parental responsibility. In effect, this means not only consent given by parents and guardians but also by a local authority under a care order. (The legal situation in Scotland is somewhat different, as is discussed in chapter 3.) Even where a refusal by a competent child or young person cannot override valid consent given by a person with parental responsibility, the fact of such a refusal is still an important consideration in making clinical judgments. Although there are no hard and fast rules, health professionals are increasingly reluctant to impose invasive treatment, even with parental consent, on competent minors who resolutely and consistently refuse it. In such circumstances, legal advice should be sought and some cases may need court review. This is more likely if the treatment is controversial in some way or the long term benefits of imposing it are in doubt.

Refusal by a child whose competence may be in doubt: Children and young people who are severely mentally ill may refuse treatment because they do not believe themselves to be ill. Negotiation with the patient is important in such cases but decisions have to be made regarding the point at which the collaborative effort can no longer be sustained. Families are also anxious that they should have an opportunity of voicing their concerns and suggestions for solutions. Good communication between the health team and people close to the patient should help avoid situations in which young patients with a mental disorder might be given autonomy in such a way as to incur harm to themselves and to other people.

The case of M

At the age of five, M was said to be hyperactive. Her parents coped with this through a programme of sports activities rather than by medication, which seemed to work well until M entered her teenage years. M was 14 when she was eventually taken into local authority care in 1989. Prior to this, she had demonstrated increasingly unpredictable, disruptive behaviour. At school, she had been prone to bouts of violence and aggression. She continued to be increasingly angry and violent. As there had been a history of behaviour problems in other family members, M's mother asked for various tests, including an electroencephalogram (EEG), to be carried out to ascertain whether there was a physiological cause. M refused to comply with such tests. Her wishes were respected and the tests were not done. She also refused to return home when given the option. M's mother believed that M was being given too much power to manipulate those around her. In her mother's words, M "changed solicitors, social workers, key workers, as and when she wanted ... M learned about sniffing, cutting herself, her rights in law ... She hospitalised herself and many members of the public ... [she] soon learned that as a minor, and particularly as a girl, she would rarely get into serious trouble for assault, criminal damage, violence". Despite a general reluctance for criminal charges against M to be instigated, by the age of 17 she was in Holloway prison. Eventually, M was sectioned under the Mental Health Act and detained in a secure psychiatric hospital. The EEG that her mother had requested years previously was eventually done and revealed an irregularity in M's brain. A year later, M was released. She registered with a doctor as a temporary patient and requested five days' prescription of Promazine, Nitrazepam and Procyclidine, which she received. She ingested most of these drugs the same day. Two weeks later, her body was found next to a motorway. Her mother published an article about the case, arguing that M had been given too much power and that because of her illness she lacked the ability to make decisions in her own interests. M's mother argued that the

---

> right of self-determination should be balanced against the right of young people like M to be protected from themselves.[10]

Authorisation by a court: Courts generally only need to be involved if the proposed procedure is controversial in some way or when consent is unavailable from either the patient or a person with parental responsibility. Where a statutory mechanism exists for providing treatment, the courts are reluctant to be involved outwith the appropriate framework. In some cases where courts have been asked to intervene to authorise treatment of young people, this could have been provided under the Mental Health Act.[11] It is often argued that where statutory provisions to authorise treatment already exist, these should be used in preference to seeking court authorisation. The Mental Health Act Code of Practice sets out some circumstances in which an application to court is likely to be needed.[12] These include cases where both the child and the parent lack the mental capacity to make the decision and where a person with parental responsibility does not appear to be acting in the child's best interests.

7.4 Overlapping legal frameworks for authorising mental health care

In English, Welsh and Northern Irish law there are some overlapping legal frameworks for authorising mental health care of children and young people against their wishes, including the Children Act, the common law and the Mental Health Act. (In Scotland, the option of a common law route to treat a young person with mental health problems is less certain. The mental health legislation may need to be invoked to treat a competent child contrary to his or her wishes. Refusal of treatment by competent young people in Scotland is discussed in section 3.2.4.)

In the late 1990s, the government stated its view that the English mental health legislation was "increasingly out of date" and needed reform.[13] An expert committee, whose 1999 report has been previously mentioned, was established to provide recommendations. In Scotland too, the Millan Committee was convened to review the Mental Health (Scotland) Act 1984. In the meantime, the interrelationships between the Children Act, Mental Health Act and the common law are complex. Although less clearly an issue in Scotland where it appears that parents and the courts cannot override a competent young person's refusal of treatment (see section 3.2.4), there is often a really fundamental choice about whether to work within the Mental Health Act or outside it. Health professionals working in this field need to be familiar with the limits and benefits of both and these are discussed further below.

Likely impact of the Human Rights Act

As is discussed throughout this book, all future legal cases and legislation will have to take account of the Human Rights Act 1998. As yet it is unclear what practical effect this will have but any future mental health reform and, in particular, statutory powers for compulsory treatment throughout the UK will have to reflect the rights of all citizens under the Human Rights Act. In January 2000, the Council of Europe published a white paper on the protection of the human rights and dignity of people suffering from mental disorder, especially those placed as involuntary patients in a psychiatric establishment.[14] Its purpose was to obtain views prior to drawing up guidelines to be included in a new Council of Europe legal instrument but the document is also likely to have a general influence on thinking in this area. In relation to the involuntary placement and treatment of children and young people, it proposed that safeguards for such patients should be at least as strong as, and ideally more stringent than, they are for adults. Building on existing international guidance, such as the Convention on Human Rights and Biomedicine,[15] the document also said in relation to consent to treatment that "the opinion of the minor shall be taken into consideration as an increasingly determining factor in proportion to his or her age and degree of maturity".[16] It also covered other rights of minors facing involuntary placement, such as the assistance of a representative from the beginning of the procedure to ensure that the minor's interests are defended and the right to residence in separate premises to those housing adults. Also mentioned is the right to educational evaluation and the provision of an individualised educational or training programme.

In daily practice, as health professionals become increasingly accustomed to integrating an awareness of the Human Rights Act into their decision making, it will become clearer whether procedures related to mental health care are challengeable under the Act. (See also chapter 6 on use of restraint.) Articles 5 and 8 of the European Convention on Human Rights, to which the Act gives force, are those most likely to impact on the care of children and young people with mental health problems. Both Articles have implications for the detention of young patients for the purposes of mental health care. Article 5 is the right to liberty and security of the person and could be invoked if arguments develop around the processes of detention under the Mental Health Act or Children Act. Article 8, the right to respect for private and family life, will be relied on when there are arguments about the informal detention of children and young people. Both Articles have been discussed by the European Court of Human Rights in Strasbourg in relation to the mental health care of a young person.[17]

Treatment of minors and the Human Rights Act

In Denmark in 1998, the mother of 12-year-old Jon Nielsen admitted him to a psychiatric hospital. The committal lasted over a period of several months and involved Jon being placed in a psychiatric ward. This was legally challenged, on the grounds that his committal to the child psychiatric ward of the state hospital constituted a deprivation of Jon's liberty under Article 5 of the European Convention on Human Rights. The court concluded, however, that Jon's hospitalisation did not amount to a deprivation of liberty within Article 5 but was a responsible exercise by his mother of her Article 8 rights in the interests of her son. Jon was described as a "normally developed 12-year-old who was capable of understanding his situation and able to express his opinion clearly".

Nielsen v Denmark

It must be noted, however, that although the *Nielsen* case is useful in showing how human rights might be invoked, it does not necessarily indicate how future cases will be decided. In fact, there are some reasons for supposing that a case with similar facts might be decided differently today in an English or Scottish court. Human rights law is a living instrument that has to be interpreted in the light of present day conditions and social attitudes. The *Nielsen* case was decided in 1998 and it can be argued that since then social attitudes towards young people's autonomy have continued to develop, especially when the young person appears competent. Views about the rights of parents to decide what should happen to their children are also changing. (In particular, see the discussion of Scottish law in chapter 3.) On the other hand, however, the principles contained in the *Nielsen* case parallel the common law principles contained in English precedents discussed in this chapter and chapter 2. On the whole, therefore, the messages we derive from the *Nielsen* case are that human rights must be interpreted in the context of current attitudes but caution is required in speculating how much the Human Rights Act will actually change the outcome of future legal cases. As is discussed in section 1.3.1, it cannot be currently assumed that the Act is automatically going to improve the rights of children and young people.

7.4.1 Treatment within the Mental Health Act or outside it: which is best?

As mentioned previously, in England, Scotland and Northern Ireland, choices are made about invoking or avoiding the Mental Health Act in the treatment of minors. In Scotland the situation appears to be that the mental health legislation would need to be invoked to provide mental health treatment to a competent child against his or her wishes. As discussed in chapter 3, the Age of Legal Capacity (Scotland) Act 1991 authorises doctors to treat competent, consenting children and young people without their parents' consent. The Millan Committee reviewing Scottish mental health legislation noted the existence of some uncertainty about whether a refusal of treatment by a competent minor would be equally respected. The Committee considered that particularly difficult questions arose in relation to treatment for mental health problems "as the illness itself may reduce the young person's ability to consent ... [and] ... there are concerns about using parental consent in such situations, as the young person may, rightly or wrongly, claim that their parents are the cause of their distress".[18] Therefore, the Committee suggested that any new Scottish legislation should make clear that where a young person appears to resist treatment for a mental disorder, the Mental Health Act rather than parental consent should be the appropriate trigger to allow the treatment to take place. This would then give the young person the benefit of the safeguards provided by the Act, including second opinions, right to appeal to the Sheriff or forum and the protective role of the Mental Welfare Commission.

Similar considerations need to be taken into account in the rest of the UK and where there are options about the legal route to follow, the benefits and drawbacks involved need careful consideration. In England and Wales, professional and academic debate has also focused on which legal route is likely to be best for children and young people. During its review of child and adolescent mental health services in the mid-1990s, the NHS Health Advisory Service noted the anxieties of health professionals about identifying the most appropriate legal framework in circumstances when it was necessary to detain a minor and require him or her to undergo medical treatment.[19] The advisory service noted that the choice to rely on the Mental Health Act, Children Act or common law powers of parents is often not easy. "Given the complex relationship between the two pieces of legislation and evolving relevant case law, it is not possible to provide other than general pointers that could usefully be taken into account by professionals when deciding which route to take".[20] In taking evidence for this book, it appeared to be the case that in the past many health professionals avoided invoking the Mental Health Act. One of the main reasons given for this was the perceived stigma attached to use of the Act. Another reason commonly given for avoiding invoking the Act was the fact that there are other options for children that do not apply to adults, namely parental consent and specific treatment orders under the Children Act. There are indications, however, that some practitioners who previously avoided the Mental Heath Act for children, now seem more ready to consider the particular advantages it offers, which, as mentioned above, have been highlighted by the Millan Committee. In addition, in practical terms, the fact that more places of detention for children have been made available in both the public and private sector has probably contributed to a rise in the use of the Act.

It may be impractical, however, to have a completely inflexible blanket rule saying that one legal path is necessarily better than another since much depends on the particular condition and the circumstances of the case. Each legal framework offers some advantages and some drawbacks. Choices have to be made on the basis of what best suits the individual child and the type of mental disorder from which the child suffers. Mental health care caters for a very wide range of disorders, from learning disorders and delays in acquiring certain skills to eating disorders, manic depression and drug-induced psychoses. For some of these disorders, use of the Mental Health Act may not be the best solution. It is seldom used, for example, in the management of learning disabled children. Nevertheless, in cases where the child's condition is one for which an adult patient would clearly be treated under the Act, there are good arguments for using it. What is certainly problematic, however, is that at present it appears to be somewhat arbitrary whether a child is detained under the mental health legislation or the provisions of the Children Act are invoked.

In deciding which legal route to take, health professionals need to:

- have a good understanding of the relevant legal provisions;
- have access to expert legal advice;
- keep in mind the importance of ensuring that the child's care is managed with clarity, consistency and within a recognisable framework; and
- attempt to use the least stigmatising and restrictive option that is consistent with the care and treatment options for that patient.

The specific purpose of the intervention needs to be evaluated. All relevant factors need to be taken into account, such as the length of time the child is likely to require treatment and detention and the seriousness of the illness. The decision about which legal measure to follow must reflect patients' needs, including the need for containment and for medical treatment of a mental disorder, and their preferences, wherever possible.

7.4.2 Advantages and drawbacks: the Children Act

Health professionals and families need to consider which legal route seems most applicable to the circumstances of the case. The main strengths of the Children Act in this context are seen in the way it particularly focuses attention on the wishes and needs of children. The guardian *ad litem* has the task of considering all the relevant factors in the child's case, including the child's level of maturity. This arguably provides a broader vision of the individual's circumstances. It may appear less stigmatising as it does not specifically refer to mental illness but its use may be seen as reflecting social and family failure. The Children Act requires the involvement of the courts whereas exercising powers afforded by the Mental Health Act is the consequence of professional judgment and does not involve court review. (The Children Act and its equivalents in other UK jurisdictions are discussed in chapters 2 and 3.)

Summary of points concerning the Children Act:

* focuses on the child's problems;
* is applicable to children who do not have a diagnosable psychiatric illness but could benefit from admission to a child psychiatric unit;
* under the Act, an independent guardian *ad litem* is appointed to ascertain the child's wishes;
* the guardian *ad litem* makes recommendations about the child's best interests;
* assessment is carried out according to a broad welfare checklist;
* perceived as potentially less stigmatising than the Mental Health Act;
* does not specifically address mental disorder;
* does not provide specific powers to enforce treatment;
* does not provide safeguards for the rights of the detained patient; and
* seen as particularly appropriate for younger children (under-12s).

In assessing the legal framework within which an individual child should be treated, the scope of the treatment needs to be taken into account. Treatment of minors may involve both detention in a secure environment and administration of medical treatment. Unlike the Mental Health Act, the Children Act does not specifically provide for a child's decision about treatment to be overridden and consent in such cases is usually sought from parents. If there is a dispute, the court can make an order specifying the steps to be taken. Although there is a range of differing views among health professionals, many see this Act as more appropriate for younger children and particularly for treatment of conditions such as eating disorders in under-12s. The Children Act also gives competent minors the right to refuse medical or psychiatric examination in limited circumstances (see sections 2.2.2 and 3.2.5). The extent of the child's scope to refuse was examined in a Welsh legal case in 1992, set out below (also discussed in section 2.2.2).[21] The case demonstrated that, in England, Wales and Northern Ireland, the limited statutory right of the child to refuse assessment under the Children Act can be overridden by a court.

South Glamorgan County Council v B

In 1989, at the age of 12, A was referred to an adolescent psychiatric unit because of persistent absence from school. In 1990, her father gave consent for A to go into care. After discharge, A was the subject of a series of interim care orders that her family eventually opposed. Although judged not to have any psychiatric abnormality, A continued to miss school. At 14, she began to show domineering behaviour, became obsessive and barricaded herself in a room. This type of behaviour continued for 11 months. A child psychiatrist found her coherent but uncooperative and recommended that A be removed and looked after in an adolescent psychiatric unit. This should be done, he said, not under the Mental Health Act but "as a child clearly beyond parental control, the Children Act 1999 is a more appropriate option".[22] A second psychiatrist visited A, concluded that her mental health was seriously at risk and recommended that A be received into a psychiatric unit "via the Mental Health Act or through the court".[23] A threatened suicide. Social workers concluded her condition was not suitable for an order to be made under the Mental Health Act and a third psychiatrist concluded she was not mentally ill. The guardian *ad litem* considered that A was beyond the control of her family and recommended a care order under the Children Act. Her father strongly opposed her being removed by force but her psychiatrist insisted she needed inpatient assessment. The local authority began proceedings that made A subject to an interim care order under the Children Act. It also asked the court for leave to remove A to a psychiatric assessment centre, using reasonable force and for A to be restrained from absconding from the unit. These requests were beyond the powers of the interim care order under the Children Act. The family's lawyer argued that a competent child (as A was judged to be) could refuse psychiatric assessment under the Children Act. The judge concluded

---

> that when other remedies within the Children Act had been exhausted, the courts could still override the refusal of a competent child.
>
> *South Glamorgan County Council v B*

There has been no comparable case in Scotland and, as noted in section 3.2.5, given criticism of this decision and the generally more empowering approach of Scots law towards young people it seems unlikely that the Scottish courts would follow suit.

7.4.3 Advantages and drawbacks: the Mental Health Act

Arguably, if mental illness is the defining issue, there is no strong reason why it should be handled differently in children from the way it is handled in adults. Although the Act is not currently child-centred, both the expert committee reviewing the legislation in England and the Millan Committee carrying out a parallel exercise in Scotland have mentioned the need for future legislation specifically to recognise the special needs of children and young people. Presently, the legislation gives minors the same rights and safeguards as adults. In the past, the Mental Health Act was rarely used for people under the age of 18[24] but this appears to be changing and the Act is sometimes used for treatment of eating disorders in older children as well as for other psychiatric conditions in this age group.

Summary of points concerning the Mental Health Act:

- authorises mental health treatment of patients of any age;
- generally perceived as more appropriate for teenagers than for younger children;
- seen as potentially appropriate for teenagers with sufficient understanding to make a decision (although it may be necessary to override that decision);
- may be appropriate if treatment involves the use of medication for an extended period, or electroconvulsive therapy (ECT);
- should be considered if the use of force is likely to be necessary to administer the treatment;
- allows patients to be legally detained for treatment, in the interests of their own health;
- it is not necessary to demonstrate a risk to their own or other people's safety;

- evidence must suggest that patients' mental health will deteriorate without treatment;
- does not give legal authority to compel treatment in the community;
- patients must have a diagnosable "mental disorder" but this is defined very widely in the Act;
- incorporates a number of safeguards for patients; and
- perceived as potentially stigmatising for patients.[25]

The Act does not give powers to treat people for a physical disorder unconnected with their mental disorder. The courts, however, have given a wide interpretation to "treatment for mental disorder". For example, it has been accepted that feeding without the patient's consent may form part of a programme of treatment for a mental disorder. Thus where a teenager refuses a life-saving treatment such as nasogastric nutrition, this could be provided under the Act. The Mental Health Act Commission publishes specific guidance on the treatment of anorexia nervosa under the Mental Health Act.[26]

Summary of guidance on treatment of anorexia under the Mental Health Act:

- Compulsory measures are often unnecessary but given the significant mortality associated with anorexia, clinicians may use the Act if the patient's life or health is at risk.
- Anorexia can fit within the definition of mental disorder in the Act.
- It is for health professionals to decide whether a particular patient should be detained under the Act and under which section.
- Where a patient is detained for assessment or treatment, the patient's consent should always be sought.
- The patient must be given sufficient information to understand the effects and risks of treatment and the alternatives.
- Treatment for a physical condition can only be given if clearly connected to the patient's mental disorder.
- Courts have accepted that feeding a patient by artificial means can be an integral part of treatment of anorexia.

The legislation provides a legal justification for both detention in hospital and compulsory treatment. It also gives children the same safeguards as are considered appropriate for adults in the same position, including restrictions on the continued use of drug treatments for detained patients without consent (see section 7.6.1) and an appeals and review system. Use of the Act is strongly advocated by some legal experts, who argue that young people are more likely to act responsibly if treated like adults and that young people who are compulsorily admitted for treatment in a psychiatric setting should be given the same rights as adults in that situation.[27]

The case of R

R was 15 years and 10 months old in 1991. She had a history of family problems and had been on the local authority's at risk register. R was received into voluntary care after a fight with her father. While in care, her mental health deteriorated and she began to have visual and auditory hallucinations. Her behaviour became more disturbed and there were worries that R might attempt suicide. A psychiatrist who examined R after an episode of increasingly paranoid and disturbed behaviour considered that R was ill enough to be sectioned under the Mental Health Act. She subsequently absconded from the care facility, returned to her parents' home and ran amok causing serious damage. She attacked her father with a hammer. The local authority obtained a place of safety order and a care order and placed R in an adolescent psychiatric unit where she was sedated with her consent. Concern grew, however, about whether R should be given compulsory medication because she was becoming increasingly defiant. Although R had previously given apparent consent to sedation, she now said she only consented because she had no choice and if she refused, she would be injected anyway. R was made a ward of court. The consultant treating R then applied for permission from the local authority to administer antipsychotic drugs as R had become extremely paranoid and hostile. R herself then telephoned the social services night duty department, alleging that the unit were trying to give her drugs that she did not need, against her will. The telephone call lasted three hours and the social worker concluded that R sounded rational and lucid and that she was not sectionable under the Mental Health Act. Therefore the local authority refused to give permission for the

---

antipsychotic drugs. The case eventually went to the Appeal Court where Lord Justice Farquharson said it was difficult to apply the *Gillick* competence criteria to a case such as this, where the child's capacity fluctuated under the impact of mental illness. The court ruled that R's refusal could be overridden because the primary duty of the court was to ensure her welfare; the relevance of whether she possessed mental capacity, according to the *Gillick* criteria, was seen as not determinative in that decision.[28]

Re R (A Minor) (Wardship: Consent to Treatment)

7.5 Practical aspects of mental health care

Multi-agency care: As with other types of care and treatment mentioned in this book, children's mental health services must be child-centred and aimed, where possible, at supporting children within their own families. Assessment of a child's needs should include consideration of both health and social care needs and also the needs of the family as a whole. Children and young people with serious emotional or mental health problems may be referred to any of a number of agencies or professionals but one person must be identified at an early stage as responsible for coordinating assessment and care planning.

Confidentiality and communication: A multi-agency response means that various services need to maintain contact and good working relationships in order to provide different facets of care. Children and their families should be given as much information as possible about the range and scope of services available to them in their locality. The decision about which agency coordinates assessment for services depends on the circumstances of the individual referral and the wishes of the patients and their parents or carers. Clearly, effective communication between agencies is essential but must be balanced with awareness of the young person's rights of confidentiality (see chapter 4).

Confidentiality and continuity of care: Concern has previously been expressed by expert groups about practices such as children's psychiatric health records being passed, without explicit consent, to adult mental health services if patients, previously seen as children, contact that service later in life.[29] The importance of awareness of a patients' past histories and of continuity of care are issues that need to be balanced with individuals' rights to privacy and to control information about themselves, wherever possible.

Appropriate accommodation: Children subject to compulsory care and treatment should be treated within an environment that is appropriate to their age and clinical need. The Mental Health Act Code of Practice states that "it is usually preferable for children admitted to hospital to be accommodated with others of their own age group in children's wards or adolescent units, separate from adults".[30] At present, however, insufficient specialist units exist for young people suffering from conditions such as eating disorders. Young people with mental illness should be treated within adolescent psychiatric units. Paediatric wards and adult psychiatric facilities are not the best environments for treatment of this patient group.

Restriction of liberty/restraint: General guidance and discussion of the ethical issues that arise in relation to restraint and restriction of liberty are covered in section 6.1.4. Consideration may need to be given to the question of formal detention under the mental health legislation and a view may need to be sought from social services to that effect.

7.6 Safeguards for particular medical treatments

Certain psychiatric treatments require special safeguards when proposed for any patient. Although the mental health legislation provides a system of statutory safeguards, some of these apply only to patients who have been formally detained under the Mental Health Act. Patients receiving treatment on a voluntary basis or as a result of parents having given consent may not receive the same legal protection. Clearly it is desirable that child patients who are detained under other legislation or de facto detained should be entitled to the same degree of protection, regardless of their legal status.

7.6.1 *Drug treatments*

Intramuscular injections of antipsychotic drugs carry significant health risks, particularly when given to a struggling patient. There is also a danger that medication may become a means to control difficult behaviour, rather than treatment. The Mental Health Act provides safeguards for children detained under the Act. Medication for a mental illness may be given without the child's consent for a period of three months, beginning when medication is first administered. After three months, apart from emergencies, medication can only routinely be given in limited circumstances. One option is for the patient to consent to receiving treatment. Alternatively, a second independent doctor must certify that the patient is either not capable of consenting validly or certify that although the patient has refused, the treatment should be given because it will alleviate or prevent a deterioration of the patient's condition. Even where a child patient has not been formally detained, it is good practice to obtain a second opinion if the patient refuses.

7.6.2 *Electroconvulsive therapy (ECT)*

It was reported in 1994 that a survey of child and adolescent units found 60 cases of young people receiving ECT over the previous decade. Yet the use of ECT for child patients is highly controversial and there have been calls for its prohibition. Except in an emergency, the provision of ECT to a detained child or young person requires the patient's valid consent or the certificate of a second-opinion-appointed doctor. In evidence to the Millan Committee, an argument was made that controversial treatments such as ECT and certain irreversible treatments should never be given to young people without their consent.[31] Although the Committee considered that there were counter-arguments for not completely excluding any treatments for any group of people, it requested that consideration be given to adding extra safeguards for children that went further than the safeguards required by the Adults with Incapacity (Scotland) Act. For example, it pointed to current good practice guidance on ECT that recommends that where the treatment is given to young people under the Mental Health Act, a third medical opinion should be provided by a consultant specialising in child and adolescent psychiatry.[32] In the BMA's view, if it is thought necessary to administer ECT to a child who is an informal patient, legal advice should be sought and the possibility of seeking court approval should be considered.

7.7 Timely access to services

One of the relatively new principles beginning to emerge in lists of ethical principles is that of reciprocity. This embodies the concept that patients have a positive right to the services they need in order to comply with their care programme. Children and young people may have a statutory entitlement to services under the Mental Health Act[33] or under the Children Act if defined as a "child in need".[34] Heightened awareness of individual rights as patients become more familiar with the implications of the Human Rights Act 1998 may contribute further to recognition of claims to services. Traditionally, mental health services have frequently been marginalised, making it difficult sometimes for patients to obtain timely access to the care they need. For young people in particular, difficulty in accessing appropriate mental health support services can have very profound consequences for their future development. A report published by the National Association for the Care and Resettlement of Offenders (NACRO) in 1999, for example, drew attention to the fact that in the UK, children and young people constitute a quarter of all known criminal offenders.[35] The report also indicated that children and young people suffering from poor health, including those with some types of mental health problems, were more likely to get drawn into crime than their peers. While acknowledging that the link between poor health and crime was a complex one, the report concluded that the factors that indicate a young person is at risk of offending overlap to a significant degree with those that predispose young people to adopt unhealthy lifestyles. Repeated surveys have shown that a large proportion of young offenders come into prison from unstable living conditions and that many have experienced homelessness, which makes access to medical care particularly difficult.[36] It would be invidious to imply that poor mental health is necessarily linked to behavioural problems and law-breaking. But it does seem that young people who are drawn into the criminal justice system or demonstrate persistent antisocial behaviour often do suffer from some mental health problems, and that they experience difficulty in obtaining appropriate care and treatment. The prevalence of psychosocial disorders in the young is growing[37] but there also appears to be an increasing tendency to criminalise difficult behaviour in the young. Experts consider that the combination of both trends means that mental health resources have to deal with a wide variety of problems, perpetuating the present thin spread of available expertise. Various commentators have also drawn attention to the fact that once involved with the criminal justice system, focus on "their offending behaviour tends to take precedence over developmental and mental health issues",[38] which may be ignored in a way that problems with physical health would not be, in the same situation.

In 1996, the Audit Commission considered some of the links between health and the cycle of antisocial behaviour in children and recommended that mental health professionals focus more on indirect work, supporting health visitors, family centres and voluntary groups when they are dealing with children whose behaviour is difficult.[39] Links were drawn between some forms of antisocial behaviour and the experience of emotional, physical or sexual abuse. Children who have experienced such problems are more likely to be caught up in the criminal justice system or be taken into local authority care where they manifest a common range of needs, frequently including emotional and mental health difficulties.

7.8 Appeals and complaints

As in all other spheres of medical practice, patients and their families need to be aware of how they can take forward an appeal or complaint. They must also be assured that their decision to do either will not adversely affect the continued provision of services. There are some specific measures relating to mental health care, such as a right of appeal by detained patients to a Mental Health Review Tribunal or a manager's review. It is the duty of the hospital or trust to ensure that patients and their families are aware of their rights in relation to these hearings. A child or young person has the same rights as other detained patients to a hearing by a Mental Health Review Tribunal.

The Mental Health Act Commission (Mental Welfare Commission in Scotland) also has a statutory role in hearing detained patients' complaints. Its function is to keep under review the operation of the Mental Health Act and to that end it will visit and meet any detained patient. It will also investigate any complaint made by, or on behalf of a detained patient. The

Mental Health Act code of practice makes clear that patients must be given basic information about the role of the Commission, about when it is due to visit the hospital or unit and about their rights to meet or complain to the Commissioners.[40]

Patients and their families should also be made aware of local mechanisms for registering any other type of complaint about the care or services provided. Complaints should be dealt with as promptly as possible by the manager or clinician in charge of the patient's care. When complaints cannot be resolved locally, patients need to have information about how to take them forward.

7.9 Summary

Summary of principles relevant to mental health care:

- care should be consensual wherever possible and respect patient autonomy;
- minors' views should always be taken into account;
- the provision of information and effective communication should be emphasised;
- all patients should be as involved as possible in developing their own care plan;
- care and treatment should be non-discriminatory and respect diversity;
- patient confidentiality should be respected on the same terms as in other areas of treatment;
- care should be provided in the least restrictive setting possible;
- treatment should involve the least possible segregation from family, friends and school;
- where possible, families should be involved in decisions about therapy;
- where patients are required to comply with a care regime, they must be provided with all the services specified in their care plan;
- informal care should be considered before recourse to compulsory care; and
- treatment should be evidence based.

References
1 Audit Commission. *Children in mind. Child and adolescent mental health services (CAMHS)*. London: Audit Commission, 1999.

MENTAL HEALTH CARE OF CHILDREN

2 Department of Health, Welsh Office. *Mental Health Act 1983 code of practice.* London: The Stationery Office, 1999. In Scotland, the equivalent legislation is the Mental Health (Scotland) Act 1984. Scottish Home and Health Department. *Mental Health (Scotland) Act 1984 code of practice.* London: HMSO, 1990. The Scottish code makes no specific reference to children unlike the 1999 English version. It is being redrafted.

3 Re MB (Medical Treatment) [1997] 2 FLR 426 at 437, [1997] 2 FCR 541, [1997] 8 Med LR 217, CA.

4 Strauss J, Ryan RM. Cognitive dysfunction in eating disorders. *International Journal of Eating Disorders* 1988;7:19—27.

5 Office for National Statistics. *Mental health of children and adolescents in Great Britain.* London: The Stationery Office, 2000.

6 Harbour A, Bailey S. Reforming the Mental Health Act: what are the implications for children? *Young Minds Magazine* 2000;45:12—14.

7 Kurtz A, Thornes R, Bailey S. Children in the criminal justice and secure care systems: how their mental health needs are met. *Journal of Adolescence* 1998;21:543—53:551.

8 Department of Health, Welsh Office. *Mental Health Act 1983 code of practice.* London: The Stationery Office, 1999: para 31.21.

9 Mental Health Act Review Expert Committee. *Review of the Mental Health Act 1983 report of the expert committee.* London: Department of Health, 1999.

10 Morgan S. At risk from themselves. *Young Minds Magazine* 1996;25:18—19.

11 Re R (A Minor) (Wardship: Consent to Treatment) [1992] Fam 11, [1991] 3 WLR 592, [1992] 1 FLR 190, CA; Re W (A Minor) (Medical Treatment: Court's Jurisdiction) [1993] Fam 64, [1992] 3 WLR 758, [1992] 4 All ER 627, CA.

12 Department of Health, Welsh Office. *Mental Health Act 1983 code of practice.* London: The Stationery Office, 1999: para 31.13.

13 Dobson F [Health Minister]. Foreword to Department of Health, Welsh Office. *Mental Health Act 1983 code of practice.* London: The Stationery Office, 1999.

14 Council of Europe. *White paper on the protection of the human rights and dignity of people suffering from mental disorder, especially those placed as involuntary patients in a psychiatric establishment.* Strasbourg: Council of Europe, 2000. (DIR/JUR(2000) 2).

15 Council of Europe. *Convention for the protection of human rights and dignity of the human being with regard to the application of biology and medicine: convention on human rights and biomedicine* (4. iv. 1997).

16 Council of Europe. *White paper on the protection of the human rights and dignity of people suffering from mental disorder, especially those placed as involuntary patients in a psychiatric establishment.* Strasbourg: Council of Europe, 2000. (DIR/JUR(2000) 2).

17 Nielsen v Denmark (1998) 11 EHRR 175.

18 Millan Committee. *Millan Committee review of the Mental Health (Scotland) Act 1984: 2nd consultation.* Edinburgh: Scottish Executive, 2000.

19 NHS Health Advisory Service. *Together we stand: child and adolescent mental health services. The commissioning, role and management of child and adolescent mental health services.* London: HMSO, 1995.

20 NHS Health Advisory Service. *Together we stand: child and adolescent mental health services. The commissioning, role and management of child and adolescent mental health services.* London: HMSO, 1995.

21 South Glamorgan CC v B, sub nom South Glamorgan CC v W and B [1993] FLR 574, [1993] 1 FCR 626, [1993] Fam Law 398.

22 South Glamorgan CC v B, sub nom South Glamorgan CC v W and B [1993] FLR 574 at 579, [1993] 1 FCR 626, [1993] Fam Law 398.

23 South Glamorgan CC v B, sub nom South Glamorgan CC v W and B [1993] FLR 574 at 580, [1993] 1 FCR 626, [1993] Fam Law 398.

24 See for example, Black D, Harris-Hendricks J, Wolkind S, eds. *Child psychiatry*

MENTAL HEALTH CARE OF CHILDREN

and the law, 3rd edition. London: Gaskell, 1998: 101.

25 Details of the Mental Health Act 1983 are likely to change as a result of lengthy government consultations and the recommendations of a government-appointed scoping group. Information about relevant developments will be put on the BMA website.

26 Mental Health Act Commission. *Guidance on the treatment of anorexia nervosa under the Mental Health Act 1983*. Nottingham: MHAC, 1999.

27 Freeman M. Removing rights from adolescents. *Adoption and fostering* 1992;**17**:14—19.

28 Re R (A Minor) (Wardship: Consent to Treatment) [1992] Fam 11, [1991] 3 WLR 592, [1992] 1 FLR 190, CA.

29 See for example the report of a working party in the Southampton and South West Health District. Southampton Community Health Service Trust & Hampshire County Council Social Services. *Children and adolescents and mental health practice handbook*. 1996.

30 Department of Health, Welsh Office. *Mental Health Act 1983 code of practice*. London: The Stationery Office, 1999: para 31.22.

31 Millan Committee. *Millan Committee review of the Mental Health (Scotland) Act 1984: 2nd consultation*. Edinburgh: Scottish Executive, 2000: para 8.36.

32 Clinical Resource and Audit Group Working Group on Mental Illness. *Electroconvulsive therapy (ECT). A good practice statement*. Edinburgh: CRAG, 1997: para 7.6.2.

33 Mental Health Act 1983 s117. Mental Health (Scotland) Act 1984 s8.

34 Children Act 1989 s17. Children (Northern Ireland) Order 1995 art 18. Children (Scotland) Act 1995 s22.

35 National Association for the Care and Resettlement of Offenders. *Children, health and crime*. London: NACRO, 1999.

36 National Association for the Care and Resettlement of Offenders. *Going straight home: a paper on homelessness and offenders*. London: NACRO, 1998.

37 Rutter MT, Smith DJ, eds. *Psychosocial disorders in young people*. Chichester: John Wiley & Sons, 1995.

38 Hindle D, Leheup R. Rethinking provision for delinquents. *Young Minds Magazine* 1998;**35**:16—18.

39 Audit Commission. *Misspent youth: young people and crime*. London: Audit Commission, 1996.

40 Department of Health, Welsh Office. *Mental Health Act 1983 code of practice*. London: The Stationery Office, 1999: para 14.5.

8: Sensitive or controversial procedures

In this chapter, consent and refusal are considered in the context of medical procedures that are either very sensitive or controversial. Treatment may fall into this category for a number of reasons, some are to do with the nature of the procedure itself and some are to do with the fact that the patient is young and may not be mature enough to make a valid choice. Parents face very difficult decisions, for example, when confronting the prospect of exposing a healthy young child to procedures such as bone marrow extraction in order to help a sibling. Some treatments, such as contraception, abortion and treatment for sexually transmitted disease, are rightly seen as sensitive and very personal matters for anyone but they raise particular concerns when the patient is very young or lacks the competence to choose. Whilst all patients facing particularly difficult treatment decisions need information and support, additional safeguards are needed when children and young people are involved.

This chapter begins by considering the ethical principles common to many types of sensitive or controversial treatments before considering examples of procedures that fall into that category. It cannot provide a comprehensive overview of all such interventions but aims to set out some general principles that can be applied in a wide range of circumstances.

8.1 General ethical issues

8.1.1 Balance and proportionality

Some procedures are controversial because they expose the

patient to risk of some kind of harm for the benefit of other people. While it is sometimes inevitable that children and young people have to undergo risks, such as those associated with anaesthesia and surgery, to benefit their own health, doubts arise if those risks are imposed on them by other people in pursuit of other goals. Adults can choose to undertake activities that risk their health for various reasons, including for the benefit of other people, but they cannot necessarily make those choices for their children. As is emphasised throughout this book, apart from babies and the very young, children can often express clear preferences and desires about what they would like to happen. Because of their dependent status within the family, however, and their desire to please or to react against adults, they are also particularly vulnerable to influence and pressure. The aim, therefore, must be to achieve balance and proportionality so that children are given the scope to act altruistically but the risk of them being used as a means to fulfil other people's goals is avoided. Consideration must also be given to factors such as the potential resentment experienced by healthy children who feel continually required to sacrifice their own preferences for the good of a sick sibling.

It is part of the basic role of health professionals to assess, when making every treatment decision, whether the risks and disadvantages of a procedure are outweighed by the anticipated gains. Where the main disadvantages are for one child and the main gains for another person, as may occur in genetic testing, paternity testing or tissue donation, this can be problematic. In such cases, health professionals have a responsibility not only to ensure that each person's rights are respected but also that an otherwise healthy person is not foreseeably harmed. The professional duty to protect the vulnerable from risks — especially if a person appears to have been given little choice in the matter — raises again the slippery question of how "harm" should be defined in this context.

8.1.2 Avoiding harm

In other publications, the BMA has discussed definitions of "harm" and the duty to prevent it, pointing out that the concept of harm is multifaceted and complex.[1] Harm is often seen as being an actual injury or impairment, whereas patients are also wronged (or harmed) if their own values are denied or if decisions about them are made without involving them and without taking account of their viewpoint.[2] Informed and competent adults may decide to risk or sacrifice some aspect of their own physical health to achieve some other goal. In order to help someone else, they may volunteer to donate bone marrow or a kidney, knowing the risks to their own health. They may donate DNA samples for genetic testing in order to help a relative, even though this might give them distressing information about themselves that they would prefer not to know. In such cases, the distress or physical risks incurred are perceived as disadvantages or harms that are justified by a much greater benefit. That benefit is not confined to the person helped but can also be seen as providing psychological satisfaction for the volunteer whose altruistic wishes have been put into effect. While mature and competent minors can also experience such psychological satisfaction and weigh it for themselves (if they have objective information and are free from family pressure) it is harder to see the benefit for very young children who are "volunteered" without their knowledge.

Harm would occur if the sort of decisions mentioned above were carried out against a donor's will. Furthermore, it would be ethically unsound to assume that, if they were able to express an opinion, all young children, unconscious patients and mentally incompetent adults would automatically volunteer for physical pain or discomfort in order to help someone else. Such decision making on behalf of those who cannot speak for themselves could also breach their human rights. On the other hand, it can be argued that it would also be wrong to assume that all individuals who cannot consent lack altruism and would not wish to help others, if they could do so at little inconvenience or risk to themselves. Therefore, while minors should not be exposed to pain or serious risk, it may be acceptable for them to undertake some procedures to benefit other people, as long as they are not opposed to doing so nor likely to suffer any serious or long term disadvantage. Furthermore, parents may be able to consent on behalf of a child who is too immature to give a view, provided the intervention is not *against* the child's interests even if it is not positively in the child's interest. The taking of blood for research may fall into this category. (But see also the discussion of venepuncture for research in chapter 9.)

Finally, on the issue of harm, the point needs to be made that although health professionals have an ethical duty to avoid harm, this obviously does not mean that only comparatively risk-free procedures can be undertaken on children for their own benefit. Where the harm is outweighed by the expected benefit for the child, interventions can be justified. Some degree of risk is both inevitable and acceptable, since every medical intervention carries some risk. (See the discussion of "acceptable risk" in section 9.6.3.) Nevertheless, we emphasise that for any controversial procedures, or where the risks are serious or unpredictable, an independent medical opinion and legal advice should be sought.

8.1.3 Confidentiality and shared decision making

Although minors have rights of confidentiality, in most cases parents are involved in decision making. This book emphasises the ideal of a supportive, tripartite partnership between the young patient, parents and health professionals. The same ideal applies to treatments that are sensitive or controversial. For patients of any age, difficult decisions about serious or controversial treatments should ideally be made with factual medical information and moral support. Family support, however, is not always available and health professionals may face dilemmas about whether the family can even be informed. (Examples of such circumstances are given below in section 8.3 and confidentiality is discussed further in chapter 4. The role of parents in Scotland to give guidance and direction is discussed in chapter 3.)

8.2 Live donation of organs and tissue

8.2.1 Assessing "benefit" and "best interests"

Whilst the concepts of benefit and best interests (see chapter 1) are the paramount criteria in decision making with children and young people, they do not necessarily prevent young children from undergoing procedures or testing to help other people. All patients' interests are multifaceted and their various physical, emotional, social and psychological needs have to be taken into account. Children's best interests are often linked to the welfare of the people who care for them (although that consideration alone may not justify an invasive or risky procedure on a healthy child). In such cases where a child is seriously ill and requires organ or tissue donation, the entire family suffers the effects of the sick child's deteriorating condition. Families with an ill child are severely disrupted. Donation may resolve these problems.[3] Nevertheless, a very careful assessment must be made of the likely effects for the donor child. Among other important factors, such as the clinical evidence of likely success, the physical and psychological risks for a healthy donor child need to be balanced against any emotional or psychological risks for that child if a sibling suffers as a result of the lack of a donor.

Thus, interventions can sometimes be justified as being in the overall interests of the donor and on the grounds that he or she would suffer distress if another family member died. One of the difficulties, however, with this argument is the lack of a clear evidence-base to support it. In relation to bone marrow donation, clear published evidence of psychological benefit to child donors is scarce and studies appear to give contradictory findings. In comparisons of paediatric donors with non-donor siblings of marrow recipients, small studies have suggested increased behavioural problems, anxiety and depression in the donors.[4] On the other hand, donors also showed more adaptive skills and fewer behavioural problems at school.[5] A pilot sample in a study published in 1996 revealed that immediately after marrow aspiration, donors perceived it in a positive light but a larger uncontrolled study found that many donors had been distressed.[6, 7] A sense of perspective and balance is essential. Studies show, for example that "many siblings of cancer patients, even where bone marrow transplant is not involved, suffer anxiety, depression, isolation and behavioural problems ... Death of a sibling with cancer may cause guilt and insomnia, depersonalisation, behavioural problems and decreased social competence".[8] All we can conclude is that, as yet, evidence of clear benefit for child donors remains incomplete. On the other hand, it is generally true that the siblings of very sick children are affected by living with the tensions and anxieties generated by that illness and, in some cases, these may be lessened by a successful transplantation.

As in all other spheres of medical decision making, the expected benefits and burdens need to be carefully weighed in each case. Where such decisions are made on behalf of incompetent children, they are likely to be ethically acceptable if it is clear that most competent people, if asked, would generally be willing to comply in similar circumstances.[9] Clearly, where the young person is competent to make a decision, his or her views should generally be respected (bearing in mind, the comments made earlier about attempting to ensure the absence of emotional pressure).

8.2.2 Bone marrow and regenerative tissue

Parents may have a difficult choice concerning how the various interests of each child can be protected where one child needs a life-saving donation and another is a potential marrow donor. While competent young people may be able to decide for themselves whether they wish to act altruistically to save the life of a sibling, the extent to which parents can do so on a child's behalf remains debatable. Good practice includes considering the need for the involvement of other agencies. At present, donation of bone marrow does not necessarily require legal review but legal advice should be sought to ensure dispassionate assessment of the case. Testing and aspiration of bone marrow involves pain and the risks associated with anaesthesia and any surgical procedure. Guidance from the World Health Organization[10] and from the Council of Europe[11] makes clear that children can donate regenerative tissue in the following circumstances:

- donation has the potential to save life;
- there is no donor who has the competence to consent;
- the recipient is a sibling;
- the donor either consents or does not object;
- valid proxy consent is available if the donor cannot consent; and
- donation of regenerative tissue by a child who lacks competence should be approved by a "competent body".

While there is no clear definition of what might be regarded as a "competent body", the clear message is that some safeguards, in addition to parental consent, are needed and an independent opinion of the kind discussed below could be helpful.

The issue of live donation of organs or non-regenerative tissue by a child or person unable to give consent has not been considered by the courts in the UK. An English court has, however, considered the donation of regenerative bone marrow by a mentally incompetent adult to her sister.[12] (There has been no similar case in Scotland.) That application for donation to go ahead was successful, based in large part on the benefits that would accrue to the mentally incompetent donor. Justice Connell said that she would receive "an emotional, psychological and social benefit from the operation and suffer minimal discomfort". He warned, however, that:

> *It is doubtful that this case would act as a useful precedent in cases where the surgery involved is more intrusive than in this case, where the evidence shows that the bone marrow harvested is speedily regenerated and that a healthy individual can donate as much as two pints with no long term consequences at all.*[13]

8.2.3 Non-regenerative tissue donation

Unlike bone marrow, the donation of non-regenerative tissue and whole organs by minors requires court approval and could only ever be considered as an extreme option of last resort. In the BMA's view, minors should not donate whole organs and only competent adults should be considered as live donors. Most people accept that there are special rights and responsibilities inherent in the family relationship but the duties are primarily those duties owed by adults to their children rather than duties owed to each other by siblings. In any such case legal advice must be sought and an application made to the court. It is unclear whether the courts would ever authorise for example, the live donation of a kidney from a child or even from a mature minor. Although the UK has not yet adopted the Council of Europe Convention on Human Rights and Biomedicine,[14] it may be worth noting that this prohibits the donation of whole organs by people who are not able to consent.

8.2.4 Seeking consent: competent minors

As is made clear above, this discussion of consent is applicable only to donation of marrow and regenerative tissue as the BMA does not consider that minors should be live donors of whole organs or non-regenerative tissue. For regenerative tissue donation, patients and their families must be given accurate and relevant information in order to give consent or to refuse. In the case of competent minors, their own consent must be sought. As with all medical interventions, information must be given to them in terms they can understand. Children and young people may find it helpful to talk to other patients of their age who have already undergone the procedures proposed. Lord Donaldson, in a case on another issue in 1992 commented that if a young person is *Gillick* competent, both the parents and the potential donor would have to give consent to donation. He added that doctors would be well advised to seek guidance from the courts as well.[15]

The most common argument put forward in support of donation by a minor is that it is the last option and that the donor benefits emotionally if the life of a sibling is saved. The donor child may, however, have mixed feelings about a sick brother or sister who is the focus of the family's attention. Children must be given appropriate opportunities to express, without feeling guilty, their own needs, as well as their fears, ambivalences or anxieties. Therefore, notwithstanding the importance of shared decision making within families, health professionals should also have an opportunity to talk privately with the young person to explore any anxieties and any intentional or unintended pressures.

The role of health professionals includes:

• ensuring that the volunteer is competent and willing;
• providing accurate information;
• minimising the risks as far as possible; and
• verifying, as far as they are able, the absence of any kind of emotional blackmail.

A major difficulty for health professionals in such cases is ensuring the genuine voluntariness of the decision; where there is any doubt, legal and other specialist advice should be sought.

8.2.5 *Parental consent*

In some cases, the child is not competent to give independent consent to the donation of regenerative tissue. (Donation of non-regenerative tissue from people who cannot consent should not be considered.) Clearly, babies and very young children are unable to give their views. As is discussed in chapters 2 and 3, the law permits a person with parental responsibility to consent to medical treatment on behalf of a young child but this does not automatically extend to procedures that are not in the child's best interests. This has been made clear in various guidelines, including guidance published by the Department of Health:

[T]hose acting for the child can only legally give their consent provided that the intervention is for the benefit of the child. If they are responsible for allowing the child to be subjected to any risk (other than one so insignificant as to be negligible) which is not for the benefit of that child, it could be said they were acting illegally.[16]

In practice, however, a very broad definition of "benefit" or "best interests" is used, reflecting the wide definition adopted in American legal cases about children's welfare in which discussion has included the benefit of maintaining family relationships. Thus, in some situations, it appears that parents can give consent to the donation of bone marrow by a child to help a sibling. While this is not physically in the interests of the donor child, it is argued that that child can benefit emotionally and psychologically from the knowledge that another family member has been helped. In practice, parents are also permitted to consent to blood tests on babies for research purposes. Again, although of no direct benefit to the child, it is justified on the grounds that there is no harm to the child and society may benefit considerably from the research. Thus, while emphasising the concepts of benefit and best interests, it is clear that these terms are not narrowly defined. Parents can expose children to some risks to help others as long as that risk is below a certain threshold (usually categorised as "minimal" or "so insignificant as to be negligible" as the Department of Health says). Nevertheless, for any procedure that is primarily intended to help another person and involves more than minimal risk for a donor child, expert legal opinion should be sought.

Desperate parents sometimes generate a new pregnancy in the hope that the future child will have compatible tissue with a sick child in the family and be able to donate. While it is understandable that families may resort to extreme measures to save a dying child, such action severely risks compromising the rights of the new child to be loved and valued for him or herself. In particular, families need to be made aware that there are very serious reservations about (even if not a clear and universal prohibition on) children donating whole organs or non-regenerative tissue.

8.2.6 The need for dispassionate assessment of risk and benefit

In most situations, parents are generally seen as being the most appropriate people to determine the overall welfare of their young children. Nevertheless, when caring for a dying child, they naturally find it extremely difficult to take a dispassionate view of a healthy child's best interests. In some cases, health professionals may also find it difficult to assess the needs of the children independently. Without such dispassionate assessment, however, there may be doubt about the lawfulness of treatment.

Some countries have instituted formal procedures, for instance in the form of child advocates or committees of experts, to weigh up the issues and protect vulnerable young people who might become tissue donors. Some use the "substituted judgment test" for decisions on behalf of very young children, seeking to reflect what the proposed donor would decide if competent. Others rely on the best interests standard, which is the one generally followed in the UK. (The notion of best interests is discussed further in chapter 1.) Some legal experts believe a child advocate system should be introduced into the UK to ensure that any decision is as objective as possible.[17] The advocate would review the relevant medical, social and psychological reports and check that no other solution were feasible, and that the risks for the donor were minimal. The advocate would also seek to ensure that the participation of competent children was the result of their own voluntary decision. On the other hand, fears have been expressed by health professionals that such a system would lead to dangerous delays in treatment. In the BMA's view delays need not be the inevitable consequence and the Association supports the Department of Health's view in relation to donation that:

> *Mechanisms to ensure that an independent view is taken of the healthy child's best interests may be valuable. Examples might include use of an assessor who is independent of the team responsible for the sick child, or consideration of the case by a Hospital Ethics Committee or other multidisciplinary Board convened for the purpose. Best practice would suggest that a ruling should be sought from the Court before undertaking the intervention. This is particularly necessary if there is doubt about the ability of the person with parental responsibility to take a dispassionate view of the best interests of the healthy child.*[18]

Summary of advice on donation by minors:

- Objective assessment of the risks and benefits is essential.
- There are very serious reservations about the use of children and young people as live donors of organs and non-regenerative tissue. Legal advice is needed.
- Donation should not be considered when the risks exceed the expected benefits for the donor child. Among the potential benefits for the donor, consideration can be given to psychological benefits or those that arise retrospectively from the knowledge that the minor has saved the life of a sibling.
- Donation should only be allowed where it is not judged to be clearly prejudicial to the long term health of the potential child donor. The long term risks to donors cannot always be adequately predicted but a cautious evaluation should be made based on the current state of medical knowledge.

8.3 Contraception, sterilisation, abortion and sexually transmitted disease

8.3.1 Contraception

In most cases, a young person's decision to embark on a sexual relationship is voluntary but in some instances the risk of abuse or exploitation requires sensitive investigation. In some cases, peer pressure is likely to be a factor in early sexual activity. The possibility of this exercising a disproportionate influence on the young person's decision can be raised, where appropriate, by health professionals advising young people.

8.3.2 Advisory role of health professionals

When young people decide to have a sexual relationship, health professionals should be able to give them frank advice, particularly information about how to minimise risks to their future health. If the patient appears too immature or lacking in understanding to provide a valid consent to the provision of contraceptive services, that should also be discussed and the health professional should explain the reason for declining to provide that service. Early unprotected sexual intercourse may increase a number of health risks, including that of HIV infection and other sexually transmitted disease. For young women, the risks include carcinoma of the cervix as well as the physical and psychological effects of pregnancy. Information about avoidance of pregnancy and sexually transmitted disease should be available for both sexes and can be supplemented by encouraging in young people a sense of responsibility with regard for their own present and future health.

Primary care health professionals, in particular, have a vital role in this matter but some young people are apprehensive about talking to their GP for fear that confidentiality will not be respected. They worry that their GP will discuss with their parents any requests for contraceptive services. A primary task, therefore, must be to educate young people about the confidentiality they can expect from their doctor (see also chapter 4).[19]

8.3.3 Young people with learning difficulties

Attitudes to the care and education of young people with learning difficulties have undergone a transformation in recent years. It is generally accepted that, if they wish to do so, these young people should be able to experience aspects of life from which they may have been protected in the past, including romantic and sexual relationships. It may be, however, that this aspect of life is something that they explore at a later stage than many of their peers since most young people with significant learning difficulties have a highly supervised life. Clearly, there is no justification for providing contraception — particularly using invasive methods — if there is no evidence that the young person is interested in an intimate relationship and there is no identifiable risk of pregnancy. Doctors consulted in relation to a request for contraception for a young person with learning difficulties need to bear in mind the points made previously concerning contraception for any minor. Also, as with any other patient, they need to ensure that any product supplied is the most appropriate for that patient's needs. Some women with learning disability can be reliable pill-takers although they may require help from their carers. Implants or other long term contraceptive methods, such as a hormonally-loaded intrauterine system, are appropriate for some patients. It is lawful to provide contraception to a young person who is incapable of consenting if a person with parental responsibility consents to the treatment, or if it is in the best interests of the patient. In cases of doubt or difficulty, doctors should consult their lawyers.

Doctors consulted for contraception must:

- consider whether the patient understands the potential risks and benefits of the treatment and the advice given;
- discuss with the patient the value of parental support. Doctors must encourage young people to inform parents of the consultation and explore the reasons if the patient is unwilling to do so. It is important for persons under 16 seeking contraceptive advice to be aware that although the doctor is obliged to discuss the value of parental support, the doctor will respect their confidentiality;
- take into account whether the patient is likely to have sexual intercourse without contraception;
- assess whether the patient's physical or mental health or both are likely to suffer if the patient does not receive contraceptive advice or treatment; and
- consider whether the patient's best interests would require the provision of contraceptive advice or treatment or both without parental consent.

8.3.4 Contraceptive sterilisation

Sterilisation is occasionally requested for young women with serious learning difficulties. Although considerably rarer, it may also be suggested as an option for a young man with learning difficulties. In such a case in 2000 the judge, Lady Justice Butler-Sloss took the opportunity to draw attention to the relevance for both sexes of taking account of the patient's fundamental human rights and the importance of judging what would be in the individual's best interests. She said that:

> With the application of the European Convention on Human Rights and Fundamental Freedoms 1950 to English domestic law imminent, the courts should be slow to take any step which might infringe the rights of those unable to speak for themselves.[20]

She went on to say that every case required an assessment and balancing exercise of the relevant factors. These factors may well be different for male and female patients but in each case the aim must be to decide what is in the best interests of the person who is unable to make the decision for himself or herself. The BMA advises that in all cases, surgical management should only be considered if less restrictive medical options are clearly inappropriate. Furthermore, because it fundamentally affects the scope of future choices, the sterilisation of minors should only proceed with the authorisation of the court (unless sterilisation is a side effect of an essential life-prolonging therapy, such as treatment for cancer).

The necessity of involving the courts in such decisions was made clear in a legal case heard in 1987,[21] and the advisability of seeking legal review remains unchanged. In the 1987 case, the House of Lords held that:

> *A decision relating to the sterilisation of a child under 18 should only be made by a High Court judge, and a doctor who performs a sterilisation operation on such a child without leave of a court exercising the wardship jurisdiction will, notwithstanding that he has the consent of the child's parents, be liable in criminal, civil or professional proceedings.*[22]

In the absence of case law in Scotland, doctors are advised to adopt the same approach and seek legal advice in these cases. The Adults with Incapacity (Scotland) Act 2000, which covers patients over 16 years of age, allows for regulations to be made to exclude specific treatments, or classes of treatment, from proxy consent provisions.[23] It is likely that contraceptive sterilisation will be one of the treatments so excluded. When available, information about developments in this area will be put on the BMA website. In April 1999, the Royal College of Obstetricians and Gynaecologists published general guidance on male and female sterilisation.[24] This sets out a series of recommendations and again emphasises that a court judgment should be sought in any case where there are doubts about patients' ability to give valid consent to a procedure that permanently removes their fertility. Sterilisation for contraceptive purposes usually involves tubal ligation in young women. Before authorising such a procedure, the court will scrutinise the reasons for the request and require evidence concerning the inappropriateness of other options. Health professionals must be able to demonstrate to the court that less invasive alternatives, such as oral, injectable or intrauterine contraception, would still be unsuitable even if the patient were given help and support. Wherever possible, the young woman's own views need to be heard. Concern is sometimes expressed that the treatment may be sought primarily for the benefit of carers rather than in the interests of the patient herself. Although attention is often drawn to the difficulty of separating out the "interests" of individuals in the family context, the court will need to be convinced that sterilisation is the best option for the young woman.

8.3.5 Surgical responses to menorrhagia

Hysterectomy may, in the past, have seemed appropriate treatment for a young person with heavy menstrual bleeding that caused severe problems. In 1991, the High Court said that doctors need not refer such cases to court if two medical practitioners were satisfied that the operation was:

- necessary for therapeutic purposes;
- in the best interests of the patient; and
- that there was no practicable less intrusive means of treating the patient's condition.[25]

In a more recent case, however, the Court of Appeal stressed that these guidelines should be strictly interpreted and any "borderline" case referred to court.[26] It is a general principle that all medical interventions for people who cannot consent should be the least invasive possible to attain the desired objective. It can be argued that in most cases, the objective of menstrual management can be achieved by lesser means than surgery. Given that evidence-based clinical guidelines examining these issues have been published by the Royal College of Obstetricians and Gynaecologists,[27] it is hard to see how doctors could now be satisfied that no less intrusive means of treatment is available. As mentioned previously, less drastic alternatives should be tried first. Oral or injectable contraception or a hormonally-loaded intrauterine device may regularise and lighten menstrual bleeding. It must also be borne in mind that most women with learning disability can manage their own menstruation with appropriate education and support. Some may need assistance from their carers. In many cases, referral to special learning disability services rather than to gynaecological services is most appropriate.

Guidance on sterilisation of young women:

- Sterilisation of a patient unable to give personal consent cannot be carried out without the prior approval of a court.

In such cases, health professionals cannot accept a parent or carer's consent but must take legal advice.

- Before any invasive options are considered, all feasible alternatives should be thoroughly explored. Treatment options recommended should be the least restrictive and always focused primarily on the patient's best interests.
- The patient should be as closely involved as possible in the decision making process. Whenever possible, information should be obtained directly from the patient.
- While bearing in mind the patient's rights of confidentiality, advice should also be sought from those who look after patients whose competence is impaired. In addition to the family, professionals such as community nurses in the learning disability services, key workers and other professional carers should be consulted to ensure that an accurate picture of the patient's needs is obtained.
- Effort should be made to make the patient as much at ease as possible. A gynaecological examination is likely to be needed to assess or eliminate the possibility of organic disease. Health professionals should make every effort to ensure that the patient understands what the examination involves and gives consent for it.

8.3.6 Abortion

Britain has the highest teenage birth rate in Europe.[28] Pregnancy in under-16s is usually not a planned event and many of the young women who become pregnant before the age of 14 or 15 have an abortion. Termination of pregnancy in England, Scotland and Wales is governed by the Abortion Act 1967 as amended by the Human Fertilisation and Embryology Act 1990.[29] Doctors in these parts of the UK are, therefore, faced with requests for a termination by young patients who are capable of consenting to that procedure and whose cases fall within the legal scope of the Abortion Act. The Act does not extend to Northern Ireland where the law on abortion is based on the Offences Against the Person Act 1861. This makes it an offence to "procure a miscarriage ... unlawfully". Nevertheless, abortion is lawful and available there in certain circumstances where the physical or mental health of the pregnant woman is thought to be at risk. In 1939, the *Bourne* case found a gynaecologist not guilty of an offence for performing an abortion on a 14-year-old who was pregnant as a result of rape.[30] In that case, it was argued that the patient's mental health would be in jeopardy if the pregnancy continued. In 1994, in the case of A, a judge confirmed that:

> *The doctor's act is lawful where the continuance of the pregnancy would adversely affect the mental or physical health of the mother ... The adverse effect must, however, be a real and serious one and it will always be a question of fact and degree whether the perceived effect of non-termination is sufficiently grave to warrant terminating the unborn child.*[31]

Some competent young women requesting abortion insist that parents must not be informed. Patients may fear, for example, that their parents will disown them or threaten them if they find out. Awareness of the potential emotional and psychological sequelae of abortion, however, makes doctors anxious about the lack of family support mechanisms for such patients. Counselling may help the patient to identify supportive adults within or outside the immediate family. Ultimately, however, a patient's request for confidentiality should not be overridden except in very exceptional cases. Examples of such cases arise where the patient is already a ward of court (where the court's permission is required, see chapter 2) or where there is evidence to indicate that the patient is being exploited or is the victim of sexual abuse. Confidentiality and disclosure of information are discussed in chapter 4.

If a competent young patient agrees to her parents being involved, their consent should also be sought to the termination. In some cases, however, parents attempt to override the consent provided by the patient herself. This was the situation in the cases of P and L.

The case of P and the limits of parents' power to refuse abortion

P was 15 and in local authority care after a conviction for theft when she gave birth to a baby boy. Soon after the baby's birth, she became pregnant again and, as with her first pregnancy, her parents refused to consent to an abortion. Part of their objection was on religious grounds since P's father was a Seventh Day Adventist. P herself wanted to terminate her second pregnancy. The local authority made P a ward of court and asked the court to

---

authorise a termination. P's father opposed this, suggesting that P should give birth and take care of the second child while he and his wife raised the first. The judge, however, concluded that the second pregnancy endangered P's mental health, impeded her schooling and endangered the future of P's existing child. She had no doubt that continuance of the pregnancy involved greater risk for P and her existing child than the risks of the termination. P's welfare, as a ward of court had to be the judge's paramount consideration and the court also had to consider the welfare of P's existing son. The judge concluded that the parents' objections did not outweigh the risks to P's mental health if the pregnancy continued. Their wishes could not "weigh in the balance against the needs of this girl so as to prevent the termination", which was ruled to be in P's best interests.[32]

Re P (A Minor)

The case of L

L was a pregnant 12-year-old who wished to have an abortion. L had been raised by her grandparents who supported her wish but L's mother, who had maintained close contact with L, did not agree and opposed an application by the local authority for L to have a termination of pregnancy. Notwithstanding the mother's objection, the judge concluded that an abortion would be in L's best interests, given her age and small build, the trauma of an unwanted pregnancy and the disruption to her education.[33]

Re B (Wardship: Abortion)

If a young pregnant person is assessed as lacking competence, a person with parental responsibility can legally consent to her undergoing a termination. In all cases, the patient's views must be heard and considered. If an incompetent minor refuses to permit parental involvement, expert legal advice should be sought. This should clarify whether the parents should be informed against her wishes. The termination cannot proceed without valid consent, except in an emergency. This may require an application to the courts. If doctors believe that the patient is insufficiently mature to consent validly to termination of pregnancy, this raises the question of whether the patient was also unable to consent to sexual intercourse. Rape is invariably a serious crime that must be investigated. The first duty of health professionals concerns the welfare of the patient who may need to be referred for specialised help.

8.3.7 Treatment for sexually transmitted disease

Sexually transmitted disease (STD) is a risk for both young men and young women. While STDs generally, and HIV specifically, present risks to all sexually active age-groups, these risks may be particularly acute for young people, some of whom may have a higher than average rate of partner change. Young people are also likely to feel less confident about insisting on safer sex practices. Evidence suggests that adolescent girls have a higher prevalence of cervical ectopy than adult women, which makes them especially vulnerable to infections such as chlamydia. This can permanently damage fertility. Young people of both sexes can benefit from confidential advice on prevention of HIV and other STDs, which can be given during consultations related to contraception or on other appropriate occasions.

Some dilemmas raised by doctors focus on the issue of confidentiality in cases where the patient may be risking his or her own health and that of other people. For example, young patients sometimes give false details and contact addresses and although testing positive for STDs, fail to turn up for the test result. Attempts at follow up are likely to entail the potential for breach of confidentiality as parents may see mail directed to patients' homes or query telephone messages. It is important, wherever possible, that these issues are broached with the young person at the time of the initial consultation or test and contingency plans made for relaying an adverse test result and treatment plan.

8.4 Genetic testing

Increasing emphasis is given to certain forms of genetic testing that can help people clarify some of their own health risks. Adults may also wish to undergo testing in order to provide information for other family members or to help them plan their family or other aspects of their lives, such as insurance risks. As mentioned at the beginning of the chapter, children should not generally be used as a means for helping other people attain their goals since, even where they are competent and appear to agree, the options for them to refuse may be limited.

There is, however, broad support for the availability of genetic testing of children in certain situations:

- diagnostic testing of symptomatic children to identify the cause of their illness;
- testing of children at risk of a disease that would regularly present in early childhood; and
- presymptomatic predictive testing to identify children who may benefit from early treatment.

Despite the fairly wide consensus on testing in these circumstances, there are other forms of genetic testing that are more controversial. Of these, debate so far has concentrated on two main areas:

- carrier testing that will only be of interest to the child when he or she is planning a family; and
- predictive genetic testing for late onset diseases where no treatment is available.

The BMA has considered these issues in some depth in its publication *Human genetics: choice and responsibility.*[34] A summary of the main points is set out below.

8.4.1 Carrier testing

Carrier testing of very young children, who are clearly not competent to give consent, raises difficult issues. Because the information has no practical relevance while the child is young and will not be utilised until some time after the child is mature enough to take control of his or her own health care, there are strong arguments for delaying testing until the child is sufficiently mature to make a personal decision. Many parents, however, wish to know whether their child is a carrier of the disorder for which the family is at risk. In reality, the interests of the child cannot be considered totally in isolation from the interests of his or her parents and other family members. Although it may appear to be contrary to the child's interests to test the child in order to relieve the concerns of the parents, health professionals recognise that family dynamics and cohesion are important to all of the individual family members and their wellbeing. Disharmony in one sphere may lead to a breakdown, or difficulties, in relationships within the family, which, in some circumstances, may be of more harm to the child than acceding to the parent's request.

With requests for carrier testing, the young child's rights to make his or her own decisions in the future, to confidentiality and to be protected from potentially harmful information appears to conflict with the parents' "right" to choose testing for their child and to make decisions that they perceive to be in their child's best interests. The BMA believes there should be a presumption against testing young children for carrier status, whilst accepting that there will be cases where testing of young children at their parents' request is the best course of action in the circumstances. In the vast majority of cases agreement to defer testing is reached after discussion between the health professionals and the parents. In the rare cases where, after discussion, such agreement cannot be reached, the benefits and harms should be considered, not to reach the "correct" answer, but to assist with balancing the conflicting interests, in order to ensure that the decision making process is transparent and the conclusion reached can be justified.

Where a young person understands the implications of carrier status and clearly consents to testing, with no suggestion that the consent is given under pressure, there are strong arguments for respecting that individual's informed choices and acceding to the request. It is clearly desirable for young people to have their parents' support for such important decisions.

8.4.2 Predictive testing for late onset disorders

Predictive testing of young children for serious late onset disorders (such as Huntington's disease) at the request of their parents is very controversial and such requests, although rare, raise serious concerns. There is general agreement that requests for this type of testing in children should be opposed because it would undermine the future adult's right to make his or her own decision about whether to be tested. The very low take-up rate among adults for predictive testing for Huntington's disease suggests that many people who know they are at risk judge that the actual or potential harms of testing outweigh the benefits. Testing children, on the basis of parental consent, denies children the opportunity to take the option that most people favour.

SENSITIVE OR CONTROVERSIAL PROCEDURES

There are also major concerns about the effect on the child of knowing that in adult life he or she will develop a severe genetic disorder and that nothing can be done to prevent it. It is feared that learning such news, in childhood or adolescence, could have a very negative effect on the individual's self esteem and ability to function properly in society. Furthermore, it has been argued that such knowledge would rob the child of a carefree childhood and put him or her under additional strain during adolescence, when pressures are already great. The child's privacy would be lost because the parents or adult requesting the test would be informed of the results. There is also a concern that those who find their children to be affected by a late onset disorder may reflect this in the way they behave towards their children, for example treating them as though they are ill before the disorder becomes manifest or failing to give them encouragement to do well at school or to train for a career. An unfavourable test result might also harm the future life opportunities for the child through disadvantage in employment and insurance.

In view of these concerns, the child's future right to make his or her own decisions must be respected. It is not appropriate to test young children for adult onset disorders, unless there is an obvious benefit to the child that clearly outweighs the disadvantages. This does not mean that the child should grow up in ignorance of the condition and, in practice, many children grow up with the knowledge that they are at risk of developing a genetic disorder.

With presymptomatic testing for adult onset disorders, where there is no medical benefit, a very high level of capacity would be expected before a young person could give a valid consent. In practice, there are likely to be very few cases where children or young people request this and have the requisite capacity to consent to presymptomatic testing. Many health professionals have serious concerns about presymptomatic testing of minors, regardless of their mental capacity and understanding. Any health professional providing presymptomatic testing to a minor must be prepared to justify that decision, on grounds of the individual's competence, and has a responsibility to ensure that he or she has been given and understood sufficient information, received extensive counselling and considered the implications of a positive test for him or herself and for other family members. The young person should also be strongly encouraged to involve his or her parents or another adult in this important decision. Before proceeding with testing, health professionals should satisfy themselves that an appropriate support mechanism is available for the young person.

8.5 Sensitive or controversial procedures required for legal reasons

Some medical examinations that lack a therapeutic purpose are carried out for purely legal reasons. Before seeking consent for the examination or test, its purpose should be clearly explained to the child, if he or she is sufficiently mature to understand, and to the parents.

8.5.1 Paternity testing

Paternity testing is usually carried out at the request of parents to clarify legal obligations for financial support but may have a lasting effect on the child's relationships with other family members. It is important that doctors try to ensure that those requesting paternity testing have thought about the potential effect the result may have on the child. The courts, however, have made it clear that determining the truth is usually best for the child.[35] Thus, the health professional's role should be to consider whether the child's and family's needs for support and counselling are met rather than refusing to assist with the test. In the provision of counselling, the child's interests as well as the adults' wishes should be taken into account.[36]

8.5.2 Assessment of age

Age assessment is also often carried out for purely legal reasons on young people applying for asylum or refugee status in the UK. If they are judged to be over the age of 18, their rights are significantly diminished. Expert medical opinion is that current methods of assessing age are not entirely reliable. Detailed guidance on this issue has been published by the Royal College of Paediatrics and Child Health together with the King's Fund.[37] In cases where their age cannot be verified, young people should be given the benefit of the doubt and given the rights accorded to minors.

8.5.3 Assessment in the case of alleged abuse

The primary consideration in the case of alleged child abuse or neglect must be the care of the child. In addition, the Crown Prosecution Service may also have an interest in clarifying whether sufficient evidence exists to mount a criminal prosecution against an alleged perpetrator. Guidance concerning the conduct of medical examinations in the course of child protection proceedings is given in appendix 1.

8.5.4 Use of covert surveillance

Video surveillance of children can be helpful in some circumstances. Patients, carers and any others who may be filmed generally need to be aware that cameras are in use for security or other purposes.

Covert surveillance, however, is sometimes used to record children receiving treatment in order to gather information for diagnosis of Munchausen's Syndrome by Proxy in carers. Such surveillance may also be used for non-diagnostic purposes, to provide evidence identifying child abuse for use in legal proceedings. As a general principle, it is essential that children are not placed at any risk, particularly if the purpose is non-diagnostic but to secure evidence for the purposes of prosecution.

In May 2000, the Griffiths Inquiry into research and other practices in the North Staffordshire Hospital NHS Trust looked at this practice, noting that such surveillance had also been undertaken previously at the Brompton Hospital, in accordance with a protocol agreed by a local Area Child Protection Committee and later adopted in North Staffordshire.[38] The inquiry recommended that the Department of Health convene an expert and multidisciplinary panel to review methods of identification of children who have had illnesses induced or fabricated by a carer. It also recommended that new guidance be produced by the Department on the use of covert video surveillance within the existing child protection guidelines.[39]

8.6 Ensuring best practice

All of the medical interventions discussed in this chapter are in some way controversial or particularly sensitive. Societal attitudes, however, evolve and change regarding what can be considered routine, what is controversial and what is an acceptable medical response to helping patients with sensitive medical conditions, such as unwanted pregnancy or sexually transmitted diseases. As we have discussed above, professional and societal views have radically altered in recent decades about interventions such as the sterilisation of young women with learning difficulties. It goes without saying that health professionals must ensure that they are familiar with new or less invasive procedures and technologies that have the potential to benefit their patients. Equally, they must keep abreast of changing attitudes that may significantly affect their areas of practice. It is important, therefore, that doctors make all reasonable effort to be familiar with good practice guidelines as they emerge. Areas of ethical uncertainty, such as those which might arise in relation to the use of procedures like covert video surveillance, may need to be brought to the attention of professional bodies and policy makers so that clear guidance can be produced to encompass newly emerging dilemmas. As is discussed further in chapter 9, doctors should also participate in appraisal, audit and external scrutiny of their practice by means of clinical governance and revalidation as further means of ensuring that their own views and practices are not seriously out of step with accepted professional standards (see section 9.6.4).

8.7 Summary

- Some treatment decisions, such as sterilisation, involving minors are so serious that the courts have said that each case should be brought before them for independent review. When faced with such cases, it is essential that health professionals seek legal advice. Although, in general, the courts have often supported the views of health professionals in a range of sensitive or controversial cases, this is not invariably so. In England and Wales, any proposal to sterilise a person under 18 requires court approval, and this is likely to be necessary in other UK jurisdictions.
- The patient's best interests are the main criteria in decision making with children and young people. Best interests should be pursued in a holistic manner, taking into account the young patient's various physical, emotional, social, cultural and psychological needs.

- Once they understand the options, patients are usually the best arbiters of their own interests. Where possible, however, decisions should ideally be family-centred.
- Legally, parents and people with parental responsibility can give proxy consent to procedures that are in the child's interests but cannot validly authorise procedures that are not in the minor's interest. If serious disputes arise in connection with controversial treatments, the courts may have to decide where the child's interests lie.
- Medical interventions may be ethically acceptable when they are neutral. That is to say, even if they are not directly in the child's own interests, they may be permissible if not clearly contrary to those best interests. Informed parental consent, and wherever possible the child's own agreement, are required in such cases.
- In the BMA's view, minors should not be donors of non-regenerative tissue or whole organs.
- Confidentiality is an important principle but is not absolute. The degree to which any patient's privacy is respected depends on the implications of doing so both for that person and for others. Establishing a trusting relationship is an important step that affects patients' long term attitudes to health professionals but secrecy cannot be promised if serious harm is likely to result.
- Views about what constitute sensitive or controversial procedures change over time. Parental consent is not always sufficient to justify an intervention that does not demonstrably appear to be in the child's own interests. If in doubt, doctors should seek legal advice.

References

1 See, for example, British Medical Association. *Medical ethics today: its practice and philosophy.* London: BMA, 1993: chapters 3, 6 and 13.
2 British Medical Association. *Medical ethics today: its practice and philosophy.* London: BMA, 1993: 77.
3 Brent KA. *Bone marrow donation by children: a challenge to the concept of informed consent* [unpublished manuscript]. London: Institute of Child Health, 2000.
4 Pot-Mees CC, Zeitlin H. Psychosocial consequences of bone marrow transplantation children: a preliminary communication. *J Psychosoc Onc* 1987;5:73—81.
5 Packman WL, Crittenden MR, Schaeffer E, Bongar B, Rieger Fischer JB, Cowan MJ. Psychosocial consequences of bone marrow transplantation in donor and non-donor siblings. *J Dev Behav Pediatr* 1997;18:244—53.
6 Weisz V, Robbenholt JK. Risks and benefits of pediatric bone marrow donation: a critical need of research. *Behaviour Sci Law* 1996;14:375—91.

SENSITIVE OR CONTROVERSIAL PROCEDURES

7 Pujo *et al.* Psychological aspects of bone marrow donation in donor brothers and sisters: a critical need of research. *Pediatrie-bucur* 1993;**48**:337—41.

8 Brent KA. *Bone marrow donation by children: a challenge to the concept of informed consent* [unpublished manuscript]. London: Institute of Child Health, 2000.

9 This argument is explored in detail in relation to genetic testing of incompetent adults in British Medical Association. *Human genetics: choice and responsibility.* Oxford: Oxford University Press, 1998.

10 World Health Organization. *Guiding principles on human organ transplantation.* Geneva: WHO, 1991.

11 Council of Europe. Resolution (78)29 on the harmonisation of legislation of member states relating to the removal, grafting and transplantation of human substances, 1978; Guidelines issued by the Third Conference of European Health Ministers, Council of Europe, Nov 1987; Convention for the Protection of Human Rights and Dignity of the Human Being with Regard to the Application of Biology and Medicine: Convention on Human Rights and Biomedicine (4. iv. 1997).

12 Re Y (Mental Patient: Bone Marrow Donation), sub nom Re Y (Mental Incapacity: Bone Marrow Transplant), Re Y (Adult Patient) (Transplant: Bone Marrow) [1997] Fam 110, [1997] 2 WLR 556, [1996] 2 FLR 787.

13 Re Y (Mental Patient: Bone Marrow Donation), sub nom Re Y (Mental Incapacity: Bone Marrow Transplant), Re Y (Adult Patient) (Transplant: Bone Marrow) [1997] Fam 110 [1997] 2 WLR 556 at 562, [1996] 2 FLR 787.

14 Convention for the Protection of Human Rights and Dignity of the Human Being with Regard to the Application of Biology and Medicine: Convention on Human Rights and Biomedicine (4. iv. 1997): Article 20.

15 Re W (A Minor) (Medical Treatment: Court's Jurisdiction) [1993] Fam 64, [1992] 3 WLR 758, [1992] 4 All ER 627, CA.

16 Department of Health. *Local research ethics committees.* London: Department of Health, 1991. (HSG (91) 5): 16.

17 Delaney L. Protecting children from forced altruism: the legal approach. *BMJ* 1996;**312**:240. Mumford SE. Donation without consent? Legal developments in bone marrow transplantation. *British Journal of Haematology* 1998;**101**:599—602.

18 Department of Health. *1999 guide to consent for examination or treatment* [consultation draft]. London: Department of Health, 1999: 16.

19 British Medical Association, Brook Advisory Centres, Family Planning Association, Health Education Authority, Royal College of General Practitioners. *Confidentiality and people under 16.* London: BMA, 1993. For advice about informing young people about their rights to confidentiality, see also British Medical Association, Brook Advisory Centres, Royal College of General Practitioners, Royal College of Nursing. *Confidentiality and young people. Improving teenagers' uptake of health advice. A toolkit for general practices.* London: Brook Advisory Centres, 2000.

20 Re A (Male Sterilisation) [2000] 1 FLR 549 at 556.

21 Re B (A Minor) (Wardship: Sterilisation) [1988] AC 199, [1987] 2 WLR 1213, [1987] 2 All ER 206, [1987] 2 FLR 314, HL.

22 Re B (A Minor) (Wardship: Sterilisation) [1988] AC 199 at 199.

23 Adults with Incapacity (Scotland) Act 2000 s45.

24 Royal College of Obstetricians and Gynaecologists. *Male and female sterilisation.* London: RCOG, 1999.

25 Re GF (Medical Treatment), sub nom Re G (Termination of Pregnancy), Re GF (A Patient) [1992] 1 FLR 293, [1991] FCR 786, [1993] 4 Med LR 77.

26 Re S (Sterilisation: Patient's Best Interests) sub nom Re SL (Adult Patient: Medical Treatment), SL v SL [2000] 1 FLR 465, [2000] 1 FCR 361, [2000] Fam Law 322.

27 Royal College of Obstetricians and Gynaecologists. *The management of menorrhagia in secondary care.* London: RCOG, 2000.

28 EUROSTAT (Statistical Office for the European Community). *A social portrait of Europe*. Luxembourg: Office for official publications of the European Community, 1991.

29 For information about the law on abortion, see *The law and ethics of abortion: BMA views*. London: BMA, 1999.

30 R v Bourne [1939] 1 KB 687.

31 Unreported case discussed in Lee S. An A to K to Z of abortion law in Northern Ireland: abortion on remand. In: Furedi A, ed. *The abortion law in Northern Ireland*. Belfast: Family Planning Association Northern Ireland, 1995.

32 Re P (A Minor) [1986] 1 FLR 272, (1981) 80 LGR 301, CA.

33 Re B (Wardship: Abortion) [1991] 2 FLR 426.

34 British Medical Association. *Human genetics: choice and responsibility*. Oxford: Oxford University Press, 1998.

35 Re H (A Minor) (Blood Tests: Parental Rights) [1997] Fam 89; [1996] 3 WLR 506, [1996] 2 FLR 65, [1996] 4 All ER 28.

36 For further information see British Medical Association. *Paternity testing*. London: BMA, 1996.

37 Royal College of Paediatrics and Child Health, King's Fund. *The health of refugee children*. London: King's Fund, 1999.

38 NHS Executive, West Midlands. *Report of a review of the research framework in North Staffordshire Hospital NHS Trust* (Griffiths Inquiry). Birmingham: NHS Executive, 2000.

39 Department of Health, Home Office, Department for Education and Employment. *Working together to safeguard children*. London: Department of Health, 1999.

9: Research and innovative treatment

This chapter begins by providing a brief overview of some of the dilemmas related to research involving children. Research overlaps with the development of new surgical and pharmaceutical interventions, frequently making the borderline between research and innovative therapy hazy. This is discussed in the second part of the chapter where attention is given to the safeguards needed prior to minors being exposed to unproven treatments.

9.1 Ethical issues in research

9.1.1 Who decides?

The whole of society benefits from medical research and has an interest in ensuring that it is carried out ethically, with safeguards to protect participants. In order for treatments to be evidence-based, objective research and evaluation are required. These activities rely on the cooperation of patients and healthy volunteers. Problematic for researchers, however, is the fact that some of the conditions that urgently require research predominantly affect sectors of the population, such as babies and young children, who are unable to consent to such involvement. This situation gives rise to dilemmas. One is whether young children and other people who cannot express their own views should be completely excluded from research, as early guidelines such as the Nuremberg Code proposed.[1] Alternatively, should proxy decision makers, normally parents, decide and if so, how can the child's interests be best protected from bad decisions when parents may be very desperate to help find a cure or if they have not received all the information they need? As is discussed further below, this was one of a number of questions raised in 2000 by a series of public inquiries into research and treatment involving children.

Other questions arise from the growing focus on individual rights, such as whether, and if so, how, the Human Rights Act 1998 will affect the involvement of children in research procedures that are not specifically designed to benefit them individually. Also, at what stage of their development should children decide for themselves about involvement in research and be able to overrule the views of parents? And, if they decide to withdraw from observational research or long term cohort studies in which they were entered when very young, can maturing children also insist on the destruction of all previous research data collected about them, even though valid parental consent was given for it at the time? While there may not be unambiguous answers to such questions, this chapter refers to published guidance and current thinking in this area.

9.1.2 "Therapeutic" and "non-therapeutic"

Since the 1960s, research has often been divided into two broad categories: "therapeutic" research, in which the pursuit of knowledge is combined with trying to improve a patient's care and "non-therapeutic", which simply aims to extend knowledge but makes no claim to benefit individual patients. While research that is combined with trying new treatment may be in the interests of a sick person because it may bring direct improvement to that patient, much research is not aimed at benefiting participants but at gaining information to help a population. Both situations can generate dilemmas. Where a child is already seriously ill, there may be a temptation to allow very risky research or innovative treatment as a desperate attempt to prolong life. When children are healthy and will gain no tangible benefit from research, questions arise as to whether parents can legally or ethically consent to interventions from which the children will derive no benefit. Accompanying the therapeutic/non-therapeutic division have been strong reservations about allowing "vulnerable" groups, such as children, to take part in projects not intended to benefit them (the non-therapeutic research projects) while there has been greater toleration of their participation in so-called therapeutic research.

Many experts now consider this categorisation to be outmoded and have suggested that the distinction should be dropped. Research guidance drawn up, for example, by the Royal College of Psychiatrists in 2000, considered such terms unhelpful and pointed out that the distinction had been criticised for excluding vulnerable patients from research and for disguising "the fact that therapeutic research (for example, a trial of a new drug) may often be considerably more hazardous than non-therapeutic research".[2] It therefore recommended dropping the distinction in favour of assessing all research according to the same criteria of risks and benefits. Other commentators have made similar points. Alderson argues that such labels can be misleading, advising that the term "therapeutic" should be abolished in this context:

"Therapeutic" is an oddly fuzzy, unscientific word; it expresses possibly unfound hopes for the future as if they were present realities, it confuses the aim of research with the activity. The word offers a licence for researchers to claim good intentions. Yet scientific rigour would assess research in terms of outcome, effectiveness and efficiency.[3]

This type of argument has increasingly influenced debate, including debate within the World Medical Association (WMA), which introduced the terminology of therapeutic/non-therapeutic into its Declaration of Helsinki in 1964. Its original intention was to allow some leeway in situations where doctors might want to modify existing treatments both to help the individual sick person and to gain better insight into what might work for other patients in that category. Research was potentially "therapeutic", in that patients for whom there was no satisfactory treatment stood a chance of improvement if their normal care were combined with new or experimental procedures. In 1998—2000, there was intense debate within the international and UK research community as the WMA discussed a major revision of the Helsinki Declaration, including the abolition of the therapeutic/non-therapeutic distinction.[4] In 2000, the WMA deleted the terms from its guidance, which it attempted also to modernise and clarify by setting out general standards for all research, at the same time insisting that extra care and safeguards should be required when any research was combined with care of the patient. In other words, it required more careful scrutiny in a range of cases including where sick people might be tempted to agree to innovative treatments and research that might conceivably benefit them, but that involve risks far beyond those a healthy person would be tempted to take. (See also section 9.6 below on innovative treatment.)

9.1.3 Concerns for vulnerable participants

The introduction of the therapeutic/non-therapeutic division resulted from long held concerns, including post-war anxiety that vulnerable people might otherwise be exploited as guinea pigs to test out new drugs or procedures. Such concerns were not entirely misplaced. Research history, since the eighteenth century when Newgate prisoners were used to test smallpox cures, contains examples of dependent people such as orphans or inmates of institutions being seen as ideal, captive (but non-consenting) research populations.[5] The Nuremberg Code of 1947 restricted participation in research to those who could give free, informed consent. This solution of excluding children completely from research, however, soon came to be seen as unjust and impractical since it meant that children would be deprived of proven treatments specifically designed to meet their requirements. This in turn could be seen as a breach of their right to the best attainable standards of health and of appropriate health care. A specific example of this issue is provided by the problem of how few drug treatments that are used with children have been tested systematically in this age group. The concern is not just about efficacy but also about possible side effects, including those that could apply to growth and development. As the Royal College of Paediatrics and Child Health says in relation to research on babies:

> It would be unethical not to do important clinical research on newborn babies and infants. To fail to do research would lead to stagnation of current practice and the continuation of medical management using untried or unproven remedies on the basis of belief rather than best evidence.[6]

Whereas in the past, and particularly in the period when the Nuremberg Code was developed, research was often seen as a potential harm from which vulnerable people should be protected, nowadays research is also seen as offering benefits to which individuals have rights. Traditionally, women of childbearing age were excluded from all research until it was recognised that this also deprived them of therapies tailored to their requirements. Social change and the long-running debate around therapies for HIV, including research on drugs to prevent mother-to-child HIV transmission in the developing world have led, in some contexts at least, to research increasingly being seen as "an opportunity or even a benefit to which people are entitled, rather than a burden from which they must be protected".[7] While it is sometimes felt that the public require persuasion about the benefits of research, particularly projects involving children, this was not the conclusion of the Griffiths Inquiry into research on treatment of babies in North Staffordshire in 2000. On the contrary, the review panel "was impressed by the attitude of many of the members of the public" and found that there was "general recognition and acceptance of the need for — and therefore the need to take part in — research of good quality".[8] Although some babies died or suffered brain damage during the course of that research, parents acknowledged the need for such investigations. Their strong protests were directed not against research as such but rather against what they perceived to be the inadequacy of the consent procedures, lack of frank discussion and apparent absence of choice regarding participation.

Thus, there appears to be some consensus that all patients, including children and babies should be eligible for inclusion in research, although the final decision about participation rests with individuals and their carers.[9] Consensus also exists about the need for clear and candid explanations of the purposes, risks and expected benefits of the research. Furthermore, it is clear that researchers should not rely on their own opinion in these areas but should ensure that the information they give is supported by independent review carried out by research ethics committees. The further questions about how children can best be protected and how much they should decide for themselves have been debated for over fifty years, as is shown by research guidelines (see section 9.1.5).

9.1.4 The ethical basis for research

The ethical basis of all research is that information gained from one patient's experience should, where feasible, be used to help others and to reduce suffering. Its purpose is to ensure that the remedies offered to patients have been appropriately tested and proven effective. Wherever possible, research should involve competent and consenting adults who have unpressured choice about participating or abstaining. Babies, children and young people should only be involved when it is essential because, for example, a particular disease only affects this group or because children might respond differently to therapies already proven effective in adults. Children and young people should also have unpressured choices.

Research on minors should not be contrary to their best interests. As a general principle, research must not disadvantage or inconvenience research subjects without their knowledge and agreement. This statement carries two implications. One is, as mentioned above, that no research can be carried out on babies, young children or incompetent adults because they cannot consent. The other is that some research may be permissible, provided that it does not disadvantage or inconvenience the incompetent subject. The majority of guidelines adopt the second approach, accepting that research that is not contrary to the interests of that person should be allowed, with suitable safeguards, even if it does not provide the individual with direct benefit.

9.1.5 Guidelines on research involving children

It is self-evident that research ethics committees (RECs) providing authorisation for, and monitoring of, research on humans must be familiar with the authoritative guidance available on that topic, as must researchers themselves. One problem, however, has been that in the late 1990s, such committees appeared to be inundated with ethical and legal guidelines. Just one REC manual[10] published in 1997, for example, contained 37 sets of national and international guidelines; fifteen of which discussed consent in relation to research on minors and two of which centred solely on children.[11] Even more guidance has been prepared since then.[12] Yet in May 2000, the Griffiths Inquiry, reviewing research procedures involving babies at the North Staffordshire Hospital NHS Trust concluded that there was still a lack of clear and "specific guidance on how valid consent is to be obtained in vulnerable groups".[13] This chapter, therefore, aims both to summarise the important points from existing guidance and to discuss some areas where gaps still remain.

9.1.6 Benefits and burdens

The Royal College of Paediatrics and Child Health (RCPCH) has published detailed advice on the involvement of children in research that points out that "[c]hildren are not small adults; they have an additional, unique set of interests".[14] Research on minors, therefore, must not only meet the minimum standards set for research on adults (well designed protocol; well conducted project; involving statistically appropriate numbers; not duplicating previous research; with external review and authorisation) but also take account of children's special interests. The RCPCH draws attention to the child's perspective:

> *Many children are vulnerable, easily bewildered and frightened, and unable to express their needs or defend their interests. Potentially with many decades ahead of them, they are likely to experience, in their development and education, the most lasting benefits or harms from research.*[15]

The importance of prior assessment of the likely benefits and burdens of research in children have been repeatedly emphasised in the literature on this subject. The RCPCH guidance includes lists of questions for researchers and RECs that should trigger debate. They are summarised below.

Assessing potential benefit of research

Magnitude of benefit

- How will the knowledge be used?
- How severe is the problem that the research seeks to alleviate?
- How common is the problem?

Probability of benefit

- How likely is the research to achieve its aims?

Beneficiaries

- Is the research intended to benefit the child participants or other children?

Resources

- Will potential benefits be limited because they are costly or require unusual expertise?

Assessment of potential burdens or harms

Types of intervention

- How invasive or intrusive is the research?

Magnitude

- How severe may the harms associated with the research be?

Probability

- How likely are the harms to occur?

Timing

- Might adverse effects be brief or lasting, immediate or delayed?

Equity

- Are a few children drawn into many projects simply because they are available?
- Are researchers relying unduly on children who already have many problems?

Interim findings

- If evidence of harm in giving or withholding certain treatment emerges during the trial, how will conflict between the interests of the child and of valid research be managed?

Views of "pain": It is clear that children should not be subject to procedures that do not benefit them and that cause pain. Opinions differ, however, about how pain should be defined. From a child's perspective, routine procedures such as venepuncture might be considered painful. Guidance from the RCPCH emphasises the diversity and unpredictability of children's responses, pointing out that procedures that do not bother one child might severely distress another.

> *Researchers sometimes underestimate high risk of pain if the effects are brief, whereas the child or parents may consider the severe transient pain is not justified by the hoped for benefit. There is evidence that tolerance of pain increases with age and maturity when the child no longer perceives medical interventions as punitive.*[16]

Because opinions differ on what is painful and where benefit outweighs the burden of pain, communication between researchers, children and their families must be very clear and explicit. As with all research, there must be proportionality: the objective must warrant the intervention. Children and families should have the opportunities to discuss their own perspective on whether the objective warrants the intervention in this individual case. In addition, research ethics committees need to consider the merits and implications of each protocol.

9.1.7 Confidentiality

All researchers need to be aware of the data protection legislation and the rights of children (and their parents in some circumstances) to access their health records (see chapter 4). Children and young people are entitled to confidentiality but it is particularly important that people close to the minor, who can protect his or her interests, are involved in the decision to participate in research. In essence, this means that parents or people with parental responsibility should be involved wherever possible. The child's own GP should also be informed. If competent young people refuse to allow parents or their GP to be informed about research projects, serious consideration needs to be given as to whether it is appropriate for them to be included. In such cases, attention needs to be given to the potential risks, firstly of the child being insufficiently supported because parents were unaware of the child's involvement in research, and secondly of a contraindicated medication being supplied by a GP who had not been told of the research. If participants are likely to wish to exclude parents and family practitioners because the research is of a particularly sensitive nature, for example, investigating teenage smoking habits, other addictions or sexual health, advice should be sought from the research ethics committee that assesses the protocol.

9.2 Types of research

9.2.1 Records-based research

Some records-based research is carried out in parallel with the provision of treatment by health professionals who already have access to the records as part of their duty of care. In such cases, where the researcher is in effect working on the data from his or her own patients, there is no breach of confidentiality as only those who already have access to the information use it for research. It must be borne in mind, however, that the use of the data in research may not be what the patient expected when it was given for treatment purposes. Clearly, the permission of patients is a prerequisite if any conclusions are published that include information about them as individuals (see chapter 4).

Much records-based research involves no contact with the patient, whose data should be anonymised to prevent identification. No disadvantage is caused to the individual whose anonymised information is used. Nevertheless, families need to be generally aware if their data are likely to be used in this way. As with all research, express authorisation for the detailed research protocol should be obtained from an appropriately constituted research ethics committee. The fact that a research project is solely records-based does not mean it is exempt from the requirement for review.

9.2.2 Research involving healthy children

The Royal College of Physicians (RCP) has provided specific advice on research on healthy volunteers that can be briefly summarised.[17] As with treatment decisions, much depends on children's capacity to make their own decisions. If children and young people have sufficient understanding and intelligence to assess the options, their view has key importance. Nevertheless, the College also recommends that even when the young person is judged competent, parental consent should also be sought for any research procedure on a healthy minor under 16. This is also advisable for young people between 16 and 18. Clearly, the duty of confidentiality owed to the young person must be taken into account but the involvement of parents or people with parental responsibility in the decision should be strongly encouraged. In such cases, details of the research, including any discomfort involved, should be explained in accessible terms to both the participant and parent. Both should sign the consent form and an objection by either should be respected.

Where children lack competence, questions arise as to whether any person, including parents, can consent in law to a child being exposed to a procedure that carries no prospect of direct benefit and some (if only minimal) risk. The RCP notes the prevailing view that, although the law on this point is somewhat unclear, the duty to act *in* the child's interests can probably be interpreted as allowing parents to agree to procedures that are not *against* those interests. (As yet, however, it is unclear how such decisions might be affected by the Human Rights Act.)

Much research on babies and young children involves relatively routine interventions such as the taking of blood samples. Where these are additional to the blood tests required for the child's own medical treatment, it is important that parents are fully aware that the samples are for research purposes and that they can refuse such use without any detriment to the child's treatment. The RCPCH has devoted much attention to blood sampling and agrees that, as far as can be currently judged, parents can consent to venepuncture for non-therapeutic purposes, as long as they have been given, and understand, a full explanation of the reasons and have balanced the risks for their child. Regarding the viewpoint of children themselves, it states:

> *Many children fear needles, but with careful explanation of the reason for venepuncture and an understanding of the effectiveness of local anaesthetic cream, they often show altruism and allow a blood sample to be taken. We believe that this has to be the child's decision. We believe that it is completely inappropriate to insist on the taking of blood for non-therapeutic reasons if a child indicates either significant unwillingness before the start of the procedure or significant stress during the procedure.*[18]

Points regarding research on healthy children and young people:

- if competent, the child must give unpressured and informed consent;
- parental consent is desirable even if the child is competent;
- parents cannot agree on a child's behalf to anything that is contrary to the child's interests (this position may be strengthened by the impact of the Human Rights Act);
- pharmacological studies on healthy children should be avoided, unless valid results can only be obtained by including children after adult studies have occurred;[19]
- there must be no financial inducement to the child or parent (expenses are permitted);

- all research projects must be carefully scrutinised by an appropriately constituted research ethics committee that considers the potential impact of the research on the research subjects.

9.2.3 Research involving sick children

One of the problems particularly highlighted by the Griffiths Inquiry in 2000 was the difficulty of obtaining valid consent for research involving clinical trials testing the appropriateness of products or procedures for vulnerable groups such as sick babies. Clearly when children are ill, the family is likely to be under physical, psychological and/or emotional stress. Some evidence given to the Inquiry reflected the view that "in some instances, no matter how often and how carefully a project was explained to a parent or research subject, it was not possible to be sure that any consent given was valid consent".[20] As a result of this and other evidence, the Inquiry recommended that professional bodies and the Department of Health should work together in producing new guidelines on consent in clinical trials. The risks of families making erroneous or premature decisions as a result of extreme anxiety and pressure is obviously something that research ethics committees and researchers need to consider when protocols involving very sick children are put forward.

The RCPCH published two separate sets of research guidance in 1999 and 2000: one on research involving babies[21] and more general guidance for research on a wider range of children.[22] In the former, it particularly recognised the pressures on parents when an infant or newborn is seriously ill and some decision about his or her treatment must be made urgently. In such cases, it suggests that a form of provisional consent or agreement in principle should be sought when health professionals are unsure what is the best option and children need treating within minutes of presentation. Various methods of resuscitating or artificially ventilating children, for example, may need to be investigated by means of a research project in order to determine the best method for a particular situation. If, however, a newborn needs to be ventilated or an infant resuscitated in an emergency, parents cannot assess in an informed way whether participation in that research project is right for their child. They could, however, agree in principle to allow health professionals to carry out one of the accepted methods in cases where there is no proven best treatment. This would permit later evaluation of the efficacy of each option. This provisional consent is discussed further below in section 9.3.2.

As with all research, approval must be obtained from a research ethics committee. Great care must be taken that a small population of children is not repeatedly called upon to participate in studies around their illness. When sick children are involved in research, it is vital that a proper explanation is given about what is entailed. Families need to understand the implications of their consent. For instance, they need to understand that by consenting to a double blind randomised trial, they have no choice regarding which treatment is given and will not even know which treatment was given, until the trial is completed. In its general guidance on research on children, the RCPCH has published a checklist of the kind of information researchers are required to give to families.

Researchers must discuss with families:

- the purpose of the research;
- whether the child stands to benefit directly and, if so, the difference between research and treatment;
- the meaning of relevant research terms (such as placebos);
- the nature of each procedure, how often or how long each may occur;
- the potential benefits and harms (both immediate and long term);
- the name of the researcher whom they can contact with enquiries;
- the name of the doctor directly responsible for the child; and
- how children can withdraw from the project.[23]

9.2.4 Psychiatric research

The Royal College of Psychiatrists has produced detailed guidance on research.[24] Its title refers specifically to psychiatric research but the actual guidance reflects good practice generally, making clear that research in this sphere must conform to the standards required for any other study. The guidance is therefore useful in other contexts as well as in guiding psychiatric research. It discusses children's and parental consent to research, urging caution in cases where parents — who are ordinarily the best judges of what is acceptable for their children — may be too ready to give assent as a result of "their fully reasonable concern to achieve a solution to the disease/disorder from which their child suffers".[25]

The guidance specifically addresses the question of whether parental consent can be overridden and the issue of disagreement about participation either between the child and parents or between the parents themselves. It concludes that when the procedures are more intrusive than those required for ordinary clinical care, a child's (verbal or non-verbal) refusal is good reason not to proceed even if parental consent has been obtained. It also urges great caution about proceeding if parents disagree about the child's participation, while recognising that there are circumstances when the consent of one parent is sufficient, for example where the child has regular contact with only one parent.

The guidance also debates the issue of evaluating risk, recommending that if the research involves risks that are greater than minimal and it cannot be carried out on consenting adults, extra advice and unambiguous support from an independent expert are essential. The guidance requires ethics committees to reject any research in which the level of risk exceeds the potential benefits in the light of all the circumstances. Where the committee estimates the risks to be acceptable, details of those risks and expected benefits must then be explained to all potential research subjects so they can make up their own minds, on an informed basis, whether they wish to participate. The guidance also strongly encourages feedback from researchers to participants on the general findings and implications of research in which they have participated.

9.2.5 Genetic research

Guidelines addressing genetic testing and screening for health care purposes and for research have been published by national and international bodies. All focus on the importance of clear, informed and free consent and also on the requirement for special safeguards for minors. The European Convention on Human Rights and Biomedicine, for example, emphasises that tests that are predictive of genetic disease may only be carried out for health purposes or for scientific research linked to health purposes, and subject to appropriate genetic counselling.[26] Particular care is needed when identifiable samples are used for genetic research that may have implications for other family members.[27]

9.2.6 Psychosocial research

Some children in clinical trials have social and clinical problems, requiring support.[28] Throughout this book, emphasis has been given to the importance of caring for the whole child within the family, involving parents wherever possible. Health professionals are generally aware of the need to engage and support the whole family when children are ill but the kinds of support that provide most benefit also need to be evaluated. The Royal College of Paediatrics and Child Health has called for more psychosocial research to be conducted to discover more about how children are affected by their experiences as patients and as research subjects.[29] Little is known about the type of support that children need in both circumstances. Such research should be conducted both independently and in conjunction with physiological research. Clearly, such research protocols should be subject — like any other research on children — to rigorous prior assessment.

9.2.7 Research involving human material

Human tissue and organs, including those from children, may be needed to assist researchers to identify the causes of childhood illness and new potential therapies. In the past, human material was sometimes retained for research purposes following coroners' postmortem examinations. In May 2000, however, the Interim Report of the Inquiry into the Management of Care of Children Receiving Complex Heart Surgery at the Bristol Royal Infirmary, was one of several reports drawing attention to the fact that parents of deceased children had often been unaware of the retention of organs. Little or no information had been given to them and even where parents had agreed to the postmortem examination itself, the Inquiry found that parents often lacked any real understanding of what was involved. The Inquiry called for a new code of practice backed with appropriate enforcement mechanisms, and identified two fundamental principles that should be prominent in retention of human material for research. "First and foremost, respect for parents and their dead child; second the value of continued access to human material for the advancement of medical care and treatment."[30]

The interim report provided some guidance itself, calling attention to the potential impact of the Human Rights Act 1998 whereby a health authority might be in breach of the law by removing, retaining or using such tissue without consulting relatives. It highlighted the possibility of a future claim arising under the Act in situations where parents discover that their children's organs had been removed without their knowledge. As the report pointed out, although the deceased child would not be considered to be a "victim" of the breach of human rights, under Article 3, the right to be free from inhuman or degrading treatment, the parents might be able to claim "that they themselves were 'victims' of the action of the relevant Health Service organisation in order to bring themselves within the ambit of the Act".[31] If the action of the health authorities caused the parents anguish and distress, such a claim might be considered valid. Article 8 protects individuals against arbitrary interference by public authorities in their private or family life. The concept of family life has been interpreted broadly but the question of whether it would include the removal, retention and use of tissue from a deceased family member has not yet been determined. A failure to seek relatives' objections could also breach the Human Tissue Act 1961.[32]

The interim report also drew attention to: the 1995 report by the Nuffield Council on Bioethics on use of human tissue;[33] the Medical Research Council's guidance on use of tissue in research;[34] guidance from the Royal College of Pathologists and the Institute of Bio-Medical Science on retention and storage of pathological records and archives,[35] and the Royal College of Pathologists' guidelines for the retention of tissues and organs.[36] Researchers in this area need to be familiar with these guidelines and, in particular, need to be aware of the need for transparency and appropriate authorisation. Discussing such issues with bereaved parents is universally acknowledged to be a difficult and challenging task that requires appropriate training. As well as being aware of the need for sensitive discussion and their responsibility to provide information, health professionals and researchers also need to consider the advisability of information leaflets. The forms authorising (a) postmortem examination and (b) retention of tissue need to be clear and to offer a range of options for which parental agreement may separately be granted or withheld. Relatives should be given their own copy of such authorisation. Also, the reports of postmortem examinations should clearly state what, if any, tissue or organs have been retained.

9.3 Consent and refusal

Information giving: An essential prerequisite for valid consent is the provision of information. Unfortunately, this requirement has not always been observed in research and even recent history is littered with examples of bad practice.[37] In 2000, one of the points to emerge from evidence collected by the Griffiths Inquiry into research involving babies was "a strong feeling of secrecy and concealment expressed by most of the interviewees. There was a general view expressed that greater openness would be beneficial to those conducting research as well as to the public".[38] The Inquiry recommended that, in addition to the individual discussions with families about details of the research and the options available, there should also be more general information available in facilities, including hospital wards, where research is conducted. Leaflets or notice boards that can be easily seen by patients and visitors could describe research taking place in the ward, describe improvements in care that have been achieved by previous research and make clear that patients are not entered into research projects without their consent. Much of the published guidance on research emphasises the value of detailed information leaflets, which can be studied at leisure, to reinforce the provision of verbal information. Written information is never a substitute, however, for thorough discussion.

9.3.1 Competent children and young people

Competent children can give ethically valid consent to participation as long as it is clear that no pressure has been put upon them to agree. Given that all research must be subject to prior review and authorisation by an ethics committee, any study that involves unacceptable risks or drawbacks should be rejected at that stage and so children should never be offered a choice that would be contrary to their interests. Nevertheless, even when the child is competent, parental consent is also desirable, particularly for younger children or procedures that carry any risk or discomfort (the legal limits of parental consent for procedures judged not to be in the child's interests are discussed below).

A fundamental ethical principle of research is that projects that could equally well be done on adults should never be done on minors. The importance of involving the research subject in the decision is emphasised in all guidelines. The European Convention on Human Rights and Biomedicine,[39] for example, requires that the individual concerned take part in the authorisation procedure as much as possible. In the case of children, it says that their opinion should be taken into consideration as an increasingly determining factor in relation to maturity and age. The clear message emerging from guidelines is that competent children should decide for themselves whether or not to participate and their view can overrule that of other people. This is probably made most explicit in the guidelines of the Royal College of Paediatrics and Child Health, which make clear that even for relatively minor procedures such as the taking of a blood sample from children "this has to be the child's decision".[40] In such cases, the evidence of significant unwillingness or significant stress would make it inappropriate to proceed.

Published guidance from a range of bodies makes the same point, namely that competent children and young people should decide for themselves and that competence is not related to age but to ability to understand and weigh the options. Most guidance, therefore, does not attempt to set an age at which children's views would be determinative (apart from emphasising the presumption of competence in over-16s) but refers to the importance of assessing competence. (An exception, however, is guidance published in 1993 by the Royal College of Nursing, which states that "the assent of children over seven years of age should usually be sought directly".[41]) The issue of children's views clashing with those of their parents is covered in the guidance drawn up by the Royal College of Psychiatrists, whose advice is mentioned above.

9.3.2 Incompetent minors/parental consent

Clearly, there has been considerable debate over the last fifty years regarding the involvement of non-autonomous people, including young children, in research. In 1999, the Royal College of Paediatrics and Child Health published specific and separate guidelines on *Safeguarding informed parental involvement in clinical research involving newborn babies and infants.*[42] While making the points that evidence-based medicine is crucial for effective patient management and that newborns and infants should not be treated on the basis of poorer quality evidence compared to other people, the guidance drew attention to anxieties about the ability of parents to consent.

"There is anxiety that at times of crisis some parents have difficulty balancing the potential risks and benefits of treatment or the pros and cons of entry to a research trial. Can consent in these instances be valid and informed?"[43] Precisely the same point subsequently arose as a recurrent theme in the review carried out by the Griffiths Inquiry into the use of continuous negative extrathoracic pressure (CNEP) in babies in North Staffordshire.[44] In that case, procedures were offered in the expectation that children would benefit as well as provide information for research. The children who participated in the Staffordshire research were very ill. In those kinds of cases, the RCPCH has suggested that consideration be given to differing stages of parental consent, consistent with the circumstances and the time available for reflection (as mentioned in section 9.2.3 above). In some types of emergency, there may be no clear best course of treatment and research required to assess which options provide maximum benefit.

Summary of RCPCH advice on parental consent to research involving sick children

- *Fully informed consent* is hard to attain in any context but is impossible in an emergency. Consent should, however, be *"sufficiently informed*, attempting to achieve the maximum level of information exchange that is realistic and reasonable in the circumstances". Parents must have balanced information and, wherever possible, time to consult friends and other advisors before deciding.
- *Informed consent* is based on a competent assessment of risks and benefits and it is essential, therefore, that the researcher makes these elements absolutely as clear as possible. Time should be allowed (24 hours where feasible) between the provision of information and decision making by the parents.
- *Consent* "comes from the exercise of choice with the consequent acceptance of partnership and involvement".
- *Provisional consent or assent* could be useful in cases where patients must be randomised within minutes of presenting (for example, research into ventilation or resuscitation in babies and children). Because of the emergency, parents lack time to assess the trial fully but may assent provisionally. Such provisional assent would need to be followed up by full information and time to consider it so that parents are in a

position to give *formal consent or refusal* if a procedure needs to be repeated or sustained over time.

- *REC approval* must consider the position carefully and specifically evaluate whether provisional consent is appropriate. (It is only appropriate where a 24-hour assimilation period is impossible.)

9.3.3 Legal aspects of parental consent

In the early 1960s, guidance from the Medical Research Council, along with that of others, drew attention to what broadly remains the strict legal position. (As mentioned previously, focus on individual rights as a result of the Human Rights Act may further bolster this position.) This guidance was reiterated in 1991:

> *It should be clearly understood that the possibility or probability that a particular investigation will be of benefit to humanity or to posterity would afford no defence in the event of legal proceedings. The individual has rights that the law protects and nobody can infringe those rights for the public good. In [non-therapeutic] investigations … it is, therefore, always necessary to ensure that the true consent of the subject is explicitly obtained. In the strict view of the law, parents and guardians of minors cannot give consent on their behalf to any procedures which are of no particular benefit to them and which may carry some risk of harm.*[45]

Subsequent to the publication of the MRC guidance, it was clarified that a person with parental responsibility can consent to an intervention that, although not in the best interests of that child, is not *against* the child's interests, for example a blood test.[46] It is now widely accepted that from an ethical perspective research can be carried out on children, when there is no expected benefit for them individually, provided there is minimal risk, strict safeguards and there is no objection from either the child or parents. Thus in 1991, the MRC revisited its earlier statement on non-therapeutic paediatric research and extended its guidance to reflect a broad consensus that children can participate in research, subject to strict safeguards.[47] When children cannot express their own views in words, researchers must recognise when a child is very upset by a procedure and accept this as a refusal. The Medical Research Council's guidance on consent in relation to children echoes the points made by a range of other reputable bodies and can be briefly summarised.

Summary of MRC guidance on consent to research on children

Research that may benefit the participant

- Minors who have sufficient understanding can consent. If over 16, parental consent is not essential but is advisable if the child's level of understanding is in doubt. If under 16, their own consent should be complemented by the consent of parents or guardians.
- Children who lack sufficient understanding can be included if parents or guardians consent and consider that the benefits outweigh the harms for that child.

Research not intended to benefit individual participants

- Competent minors can consent but it would also be prudent to have the consent of parents or guardians.
- Minors who cannot consent can be included in such research, subject to safeguards and where they are not placed at more than negligible risk of harm.
- In that case, parents or guardians must consent and agree that there is no more than negligible risk.
- The REC should consider the likely risk, which should be no more than the discomfort encountered in daily life or during routine examinations.[48]

9.4 Safeguards

Key safeguards are the provision of proper information to participants and/or their parents, and effective monitoring and audit of research by independent bodies. Some published research guidelines, such as those of the RCPCH on research on babies and infants, go into some detail about the kind of information that should be included in parent information sheets. In addition to information about the purposes, benefits and risks, of particular importance is the fact that participation is voluntary. Parents and children need to be aware that they are not obliged to participate and can withdraw at any time.

9.4.1 Governance and monitoring of research

In addition to scrutiny by ethics committees, attention has also been drawn to the need for other review. The process of external peer review, for example, is generally applied by all major medical research funding bodies. The RCPCH also makes the point that:

> As assessment of benefit and harm is complex, children are best protected if projects are reviewed at many levels, by researchers, funding and scientific bodies, research ethics committees, the research assistants and nurses working with child subjects, the children, and their parents. Everyone concerned (except young children) has some responsibility.[49]

9.4.2 Continuing review

The point has already been made that all research requires scrutiny by an appropriately constituted research ethics committee. The duties of committee members and the factors they must consider are set out in guidance from a range of reputable bodies, including the Department of Health[50] and the Royal College of Physicians.[51] Much existing guidance focuses on the initial review of the research protocol prior to its implementation. Increasingly, however, attention is moving to the way in which research should be continually monitored. One of the issues picked up by the Griffiths Inquiry, for example, was the role of research ethics committees in reviewing their past decisions and actions. In addition, the Inquiry noted the responsibility of such committees to ensure that good supervision and management processes are built into research proposals. The absence of clear guidelines about whose duty it is to ensure that research proceeds as planned, or to whom any breaches of the original protocol should be reported, were important gaps identified by the Inquiry.

Submissions to the Griffiths Inquiry on research governance included a series of recommendations from the RCPCH president, the late Professor David Baum, who set out some benchmarks of good practice.[52]

- All research should be recorded in individual log books, which should include details of the research, achievement of process targets as well as research targets, and specified responsibilities of the researchers. The log book should be in the public domain.

- The senior academic or consultant who is conducting the research, or in whose name the research is being conducted, should maintain a personal responsibility for the supervision and management of the project.
- Research projects should be subjected to rigorous scientific evaluation and, in all but the most simple projects, be subjected to external peer review.
- A culture of routine self audit should be developed among research teams.
- There was a need to balance the enthusiasm of researchers with the observance of proper process whilst avoiding unnecessary obstruction of legitimate research.
- Researchers should receive induction training on the proper conduct of research. Consideration should be given to the use of independent third parties to obtain consent to research, particularly where this involves vulnerable groups of patients or especially stressful situations where anxious patients and/or relatives might rely too heavily on medical staff.

9.4.3 Reporting and investigating adverse incidents

Adverse or unexpected incidents should be reported to the authorising research ethics committee so that it can assess whether these are significant and require the halting of the research. Systems are in place for the reporting of adverse incidents in clinical trials on drugs. One of the anxieties expressed by the Griffiths Inquiry concerning research on babies was the absence of any clear procedure for reporting adverse events where medical devices were concerned. It noted that there are no comprehensive national or regional systems for surveillance of unexpected outcomes of non-drug treatments. Clearly, there should be such a procedure in place. In studies involving very sick babies and children, there is always the prospect that the child may die or suffer disability as a result of the illness, unconnected with the actual research. Nevertheless, it is essential that such cases — even if not unexpected — are thoroughly investigated, ideally by two independent doctors in each case. (Clearly, when an unexpected death occurs, it must be reported to the coroner.)

9.4.4 Children's safety in relation to researchers

Guidance from the Royal College of Psychiatrists also considers aspects of safety in relation to the participation of children in research emphasising, for example, that there should be a police check on the records of all researchers working directly with children to reveal whether there is any history of crimes relating to minors. In the past, researchers working with charities or employed by the Medical Research Council have not been obliged to undergo such checks, which are required for those employed by universities or the NHS. The guidance acknowledges that the screening provided by checks is imperfect but maintains it is still better than nothing and therefore should be mandatory for all researchers prior to starting work with children.

9.5 The boundary between treatment and research

Unusual treatments frequently involve some element of research even though this is not the main goal of modifying a standard procedure. Consent to treatment, however, must be kept separate from the consent to the treatment being monitored for research purposes. Where the monitoring simply involves the recording of information that would be collected in any case during the course of treatment, this clearly has fewer implications. Nevertheless, the family should be kept aware that information gained from the treatment may, in an anonymised form, help inform others in the same situation.

As with research, new treatments should be tested on willing adults first wherever possible. Time also needs to be spent in assessing the outcomes for adults prior to offering the procedure to children. Obviously, there needs to be careful advance risk assessment. As the Royal College of Paediatrics and Child Health stresses:

> *The urgent desire to offer babies and children the potential benefits of medical innovation is laudable. Yet childhood is a vulnerable, formative time, when harms can have serious impact as well as being potentially long lasting.*[53]

The urgent desire to extend practice that the researcher or treating doctor believes to be beneficial was an issue identified by the Griffiths Inquiry in 2000 as one of the "potential pitfalls of human behaviour".[54] The Inquiry report drew attention to the need for caution and independent external review before instituting new procedures as routine practice and mentioned the importance of recognising the danger of bias by an enthusiastic, highly motivated researcher or practitioner. Any project that is on the boundary between research and treatment should be submitted to a research ethics committee for consideration.

9.6 Innovative treatment

As a general principle, children and young people should not be put forward for innovative treatment that involves an unknown risk and that has not previously been tested on informed adults. Generally, children should only be offered new forms of treatment once the safety and the benefit have been proven in treatment of adults. Exceptions, however, may occur in situations where there is evidence to suppose that the child's chances of recovery with treatment are better than those of an adult with a comparable condition. In extremely serious situations, therefore, where the child's health is already at grave risk and few other options are available, there may be greater willingness to undertake risks on the basis that there is little to lose but potentially much to gain. It is essential, however, that families and the health care team give careful consideration to all the known facts and avoid exposing very sick children to unproven treatments where there is significant doubt about the likelihood of success.

9.6.1 The duty of candour

By their nature, innovative treatments have less evidential support than conventional regimes. The benefit for the patient is harder to predict. At the same time, there is likely to be an intuitive wish to try anything that might help save or improve a child's life. Clinicians may be more tempted to be over-optimistic and to recommend treatment where perhaps they would not, for an older person who had already lived a long life. Parents and the patient often find it very hard to resist agreeing to any therapy — even unproven treatment — that doctors recommend.

9.6.2 The value of a second opinion

It is essential that clinicians make clear which aspects of treatment are innovative so that the family can assess the proposal in the light of that knowledge. If the treatment involves significant risk to the child, an independent and objective second opinion should always be sought before presenting the option to the family. This means that the clinician can be more confident that he or she is not putting too positive a gloss on it when explaining the option to the family. When the new treatment is invasive, the procedure for obtaining informed consent must reflect the gravity of that. Families should be fully informed if a particular practitioner or hospital introduces, on a routine basis, procedures that are not standard treatment in other facilities. It is no longer ethically acceptable for a department to rely on the concept of implied consent on the grounds that an innovative treatment is "standard" when this is plainly not a widely shared view. Families should be aware of all the options open to them even if this involves referral to another facility. Consent can never be implied or taken for granted in this situation.

9.6.3 The concept of "acceptable risk"

Assessment of risk is an important part of decision making in all forms of health care. Risk has to be assessed both in terms of the likely effects of the new procedure but also with the knowledge of the risks to the patient if it is not carried out. In other words, risk is relative rather than absolute. The degree of risk undertaken should be in proportion to the expected benefit. Assessment of risk is not limited to consideration of the particular study under discussion but must also take account of the background context in which it is likely to be implemented. The risks for participants' exposure to x-rays, for example, may differ if the child is involved in a series of studies rather than just one.

Health professionals are sometimes criticised for apparently poor communication in some situations of this type where parents have not been provided with an adequate explanation and details of the choices available.[55] Clearly, information and advice to families must also be as objective and consistent as possible with recognition given to the fact that they are faced with decisions at what is often a time of great anxiety and stress. One of the issues about which families most often seek reassurance is how much risk of harm is likely to be involved. Despite the existence of some guidelines, no generally applicable categorisation of "risk" has yet been achieved and the question of significant risk needs to be discussed on a case-by-case basis.

9.6.4 Surveillance of outcomes

As a general principle, all doctors must be assiduous in monitoring outcomes from their treatment patterns and must investigate the reasons if their success rates fall below those achieved by other practitioners in similar circumstances. The emphasis on such self monitoring and peer review is increasing. Part of the revalidation process that the statutory body for medicine, the General Medical Council (GMC), proposes to bring in will require every registered doctor, in whatever field of practice, to maintain a revalidation folder. Among other information, it is expected that this will include the results of audit and a record of the doctor's strengths or potential areas of weakness. All doctors should participate in audit initiatives. Clinicians have always modified standard treatments in individual cases where they have reason to believe that a particular patient is likely to thrive better under a different regime. It is essential, however, that the outcome from such modifications is also carefully monitored and recorded. If success rates appear consistently better with a modified procedure, a formal research protocol should be drawn up for appraisal by a research ethics committee and the innovative treatment put to the test.

9.6.5 The medical duty to act only within one's sphere of competence

As with non-controversial areas of treatment, doctors should not exceed their own knowledge and competence. Clearly, innovative medical and surgical techniques are constantly being developed and it is important that specialists are able to provide those of proven benefit and adapt them, where necessary, for children and babies. Equally clearly, however, it is unethical for doctors, who may be on a steep learning curve, to fail to monitor their own mastery of the new technique and their own success rate in performing it in comparison with national rates or those of colleagues. Regular appraisal, audit and external scrutiny by means of clinical governance and revalidation make it less likely that serious errors in practice will remain undetected. The GMC's revalidation process, mentioned above, will also keep a record of doctors' continuing professional development.

Doctors also risk exceeding their competence if they offer to provide, on another professional's recommendation, a category of care or treatment with which they themselves are unfamiliar. General practitioners, for example, are sometimes asked to prescribe and monitor new drugs that require specialist knowledge. They sometimes feel pressured to prescribe products unfamiliar to them that have a range of potential side effects. Both the BMA and the General Medical Council emphasise the ethical duty of doctors to provide only those treatments that are within their own sphere of competence.

Innovative therapy and child B[56]

B, who was 10 years old, suffered from non-Hodgkin lymphoma with common acute lymphoblastic leukaemia. In December 1993, she was diagnosed with acute myeloid leukaemia and after a variety of treatments, including chemotherapy and a bone marrow transplant, B was only given six to eight weeks to live. In January 1995, B's doctors maintained that B should be given palliative care to enable her to enjoy a normal life during her remaining weeks. American specialists consulted by B's father, however, estimated that a further two stages of treatment were possible, both of which had a 10—20% chance of success: the second stage being contingent on the first succeeding. B's father asked the health authority to allocate the £75,000 necessary to purchase this treatment. The authority refused on three grounds: (i) the clinical opinion of B's usual health care team was that the treatment was not in her best interests; (ii) the treatment was non-proven, experimental and had never been formally evaluated; (iii) the treatment was not an equitable or effective use of resources given the small prospect of success. Although when the initial case went to judicial review and to the Court of Appeal, much of the discussion concerned the expenditure involved, the fact that the treatment was, as Sir Thomas Bingham termed it, "on the frontier of medical science" without "a well-tried track record of success" also played a part in deliberations. Evidence in the Court of Appeal focused also on the view of the specialist who had cared for B since the child was five that "it would not be right to subject B to all this suffering and trauma when the prospects for success were so slight". In the event, private funding was found for B's treatment

---

but the controversy continued. B died in May 1996 at the age of 11. The doctors who treated her at the end of her life considered that the new technique had given her a few extra months of reasonably good quality life. The case "came to epitomise the dilemmas involved in making tragic choices in health care, particularly those involving individuals with life-threatening illnesses".[57]

R v Cambridge HA ex parte B

9.7 Summary

9.7.1 Summary of guidance on paediatric research

- Research should only involve children where this is essential and where the information cannot be obtained using adult volunteers.
- All projects must have REC authorisation.
- Competent children must be willing and informed before they can be included.
- Parents should be involved in the decision wherever possible.
- Research involves partnership with the child and/or family, who should be kept informed and consent to each separate stage of the project.
- Researchers must take account of the cumulative medical, emotional, social and psychological consequences of the child being involved. Children with some conditions may be exposed to a sequence of research projects. It is insufficient to consider only the risks of a particular research procedure without considering the background context and whether the child has been involved in multiple projects by different researchers.
- Researchers should be aware of the possibility of the procedures giving rise to emotional or behavioural disturbances in the child and deal with any such disturbance by prompt and appropriate referral.
- Research workers must recognise when a child is very upset by a procedure and accept this as a valid refusal.
- Researchers should be aware (and attempt to avoid) any pressures that might lead the child to volunteer for research or which might lead parents to volunteer their children, in the expectation of direct benefit (whether therapeutic or financial).

9.7.2 Summary of innovative treatment

- Doctors must monitor closely whether the outcomes from new procedures and from their mastery of them fall below the success rate gained by other practitioners. If so, attention needs to be given urgently to investigating the reasons for this.

- Where doctors modify a standard procedure or introduce a new treatment, they should inform patients and their parents of the reasons and whether there are foreseeable variations in the risks involved. Once success rates of a new procedure appear hopeful, a formal research protocol should be drawn up for appraisal by a research ethics committee. Doctors should not continue indefinitely with an innovative procedure that has not been tested against standard options.

References

1 The Nuremberg Code of 1947, which set down guidance on research, stressed the necessity of voluntary consent by the participant, emphasising that "This means that the person involved should have legal capacity to give consent; should be so situated as to be able to exercise free power of choice".

2 Royal College of Psychiatrists. *Guidelines for researchers and for ethics committees on psychiatric research involving human participants*. London: RCPsych, in press: section 3.4.

3 Alderson P. Did children change, or the guidelines? *Bulletin of Medical Ethics* 1999;**150**:38—44:40.

4 European Forum for Good Clinical Practice, Bulletin of Medical Ethics. Revising the Declaration of Helsinki: a fresh start, London, 3—4 September 1999. The findings of this international discussion were submitted to the World Medical Association.

5 See, for example, British Medical Association. *The medical profession & human rights: handbook for a changing agenda*. London: Zed Books, in press: chapter 9; Doyal L, Tobias J (eds). *Informed consent in medical research*. London: BMJ Books, 2001.

6 Royal College of Paediatrics and Child Health. *Safeguarding informed parental involvement in clinical research involving newborn babies and infants*. London: RCPCH, 1999: 2.

7 Grady C. *Review of the search for an AIDS vaccine: ethical issues in the development and testing of a preventive HIV vaccine*. Indiana: Indiana University Press, 1995.

8 NHS Executive, West Midlands. *Report of a review of the research framework in North Staffordshire Hospital NHS Trust* (Griffiths Inquiry). Birmingham: NHS Executive, 2000: para 4.2.1.

9 The ethical arguments for including children in research are explored in a number of published guidelines. See, for example, Medical Research Council. *The ethical conduct of research on children*. London: MRC, 1991.

10 *Manual for research ethics committees*, 5th edition. London: Centre of Medical Law and Ethics, King's College, London, 1997.

11 Medical Research Council. *The ethical conduct of research on children*, London: MRC, 1991; British Paediatric Association. *Guidelines for the ethical conduct of medical research involving children*. London: BPA, 1992. (The BPA subsequently became the Royal College of Paediatrics and Child Health and issued revised guidelines with the same title in 2000.)

12 Royal College of Pathologists. *Guidelines for the retention of tissues and organs at post-mortem examination*. London: RCPath, 2000; Medical Research Council. *Human tissue and biological samples for use in research. Report of the Medical Research Council working group to develop operational and ethical guidelines*. London: MRC, 1999.

13 NHS Executive, West Midlands. *Report of a review of the research framework in North Staffordshire Hospital NHS Trust* (Griffiths Inquiry). Birmingham: NHS Executive, 2000: para 6.9.8.

14 Royal College of Paediatrics and Child Health. Guidelines for the ethical conduct of medical research involving children. *Archives of Disease in Childhood* 2000;**82**:177—82:177.

15 Ibid.

16 Royal College of Paediatrics and Child Health. Guidelines for the ethical conduct of medical research involving children. *Archives of Disease in Childhood* 2000;**82**:177—82:178—9.

17 Royal College of Physicians. *Research on healthy volunteers*. London: RCP, 1986.

18 Royal College of Paediatrics and Child Health. Guidelines for the ethical conduct of medical research involving children. *Archives of Disease in Childhood* 2000;**82**:177—82:179.

19 Royal College of Physicians. *Research on healthy volunteers*. London: RCP, 1986.

20 NHS Executive, West Midlands. *Report of a review of the research framework in North Staffordshire Hospital NHS Trust* (Griffiths Inquiry). Birmingham: NHS Executive, 2000: para 4.2.2.

21 Royal College of Paediatrics and Child Health. *Safeguarding informed parental involvement in clinical research involving newborn babies and infants*. London: RCPCH, 1999.

22 Royal College of Paediatrics and Child Health. Guidelines for the ethical conduct of medical research involving children. *Archives of Disease in Childhood* 2000;**82**:177—82.

23 Royal College of Paediatrics and Child Health. Guidelines for the ethical conduct of medical research involving children. *Archives of Disease in Childhood* 2000;**82**:177—82:180—1.

24 Royal College of Psychiatrists. *Guidelines for researchers and for ethics committees on psychiatric research involving human participants*. London: RCPsych, in press.

25 Royal College of Psychiatrists. *Guidelines for researchers and for ethics committees on psychiatric research involving human participants*. London: RCPsych, in press: section 5.6a.

26 Convention for the Protection of Human Rights and Dignity of the Human Being with regard to the Application of Biology and Medicine: Convention on Human Rights and Biomedicine (4. iv. 1997): Article 12.

27 These issues are discussed in British Medical Association. *Human genetics: choice and responsibility*. Oxford: Oxford University Press, 1998.

28 Kinmonth A, Lindsay M, Baum J. Social and emotional complications: a clinical trial among adolescents with diabetes mellitus. *BMJ* 1983;**286**:952—4.

29 Royal College of Paediatrics and Child Health. Guidelines for the ethical conduct of medical research involving children. *Archives of Disease in Childhood* 2000;**82**:177—82.

30 The Bristol Royal Infirmary Inquiry. *The inquiry into the management of care of children receiving complex heart surgery at The Bristol Royal Infirmary. Interim report: removal and retention of human material*. 2000.

31 The Bristol Royal Infirmary Inquiry. *The inquiry into the management of care of children receiving complex heart surgery at The Bristol Royal Infirmary. Interim report: removal and retention of human material*. 2000: 85.

32 Human Tissue Act 1961 s1(2).

33 Nuffield Council on Bioethics. *Human tissue: ethical and legal issues*. London: Nuffield Council on Bioethics, 1995.

RESEARCH AND INNOVATIVE TREATMENT

34 Medical Research Council. *Human tissue and biological samples for use in research. Report of the Medical Research Council working group to develop operational and ethical guidelines.* London: MRC, 1999.

35 Royal College of Pathologists, Institute of Bio-Medical Science. *Consensus statement of recommended policies for uses of human tissue in research, education and quality control. With notes reflecting UK law and practices prepared by a working party of the Royal College of Pathologists and the Institute of Bio-medical Science.* London: RCPath, 1999.

36 Royal College of Pathologists. *Guidelines for the retention of tissues and organs at post-mortem examination.* London: RCPath, 2000.

37 See, for example, Doyal L, Tobias J (eds) *Informed consent in medical research.* London: BMJ Books, 2001.

38 NHS Executive, West Midlands. *Report of a review of the research framework in North Staffordshire Hospital NHS Trust* (Griffiths Inquiry). Birmingham: NHS Executive, 2000: para 10.5.2.

39 Convention for the Protection of Human Rights and Dignity of the Human Being with Regard to the Application of Biology and Medicine: Convention on Human Rights and Biomedicine (4. iv. 1997).

40 Royal College of Paediatrics and Child Health. Guidelines for the ethical conduct of medical research involving children. *Archives of Disease in Childhood* 2000;**82**:177—82:179.

41 Royal College of Nursing. *Ethics related to research in nursing.* London: RCN, 1993.

42 Royal College of Paediatrics and Child Health. *Safeguarding informed parental involvement in clinical research involving newborn babies and infants.* London: RCPCH, 1999.

43 Royal College of Paediatrics and Child Health. *Safeguarding informed parental involvement in clinical research involving newborn babies and infants.* London: RCPCH, 1999: 2.

44 NHS Executive, West Midlands. *Report of a review of the research framework in North Staffordshire Hospital NHS Trust* (Griffiths Inquiry). Birmingham: NHS Executive, 2000.

45 Medical Research Council. *The ethical conduct of research on children.* London: MRC, 1991: para 4.4.

46 S v McC (orse. S) & M (D.S. Intervener); W v W [1972] AC 24, [1970] 3 WLR 366, [1970] 3 All ER 107, HL.

47 Medical Research Council guidance on this issue closely echoes those of other responsible bodies, including the Department of Health.

48 Medical Research Council. *The ethical conduct of research on children.* London: MRC, 1991.

49 Royal College of Paediatrics and Child Health. Guidelines for the ethical conduct of medical research involving children. *Archives of Disease in Childhood* 2000;**82**:177—82:179.

50 Department of Health. *Local research ethics committees.* London: Department of Health, 1991. (HSG (91) 5).

51 Royal College of Physicians. *Guidelines on the practice of ethics committees in medical research involving human subjects.* London: RCP, 1996.

52 NHS Executive, West Midlands. *Report of a review of the research framework in North Staffordshire Hospital NHS Trust* (Griffiths Inquiry). Birmingham: NHS Executive, 2000: para 15.2.1. Evidence put forward by the late Professor David Baum.

53 Royal College of Paediatrics and Child Health. Guidelines for the ethical conduct of medical research involving children. *Archives of Disease in Childhood* 2000;**82**:177—82:178.

54 NHS Executive, West Midlands. *Report of a review of the research framework in North Staffordshire Hospital NHS Trust* (Griffiths Inquiry). Birmingham: NHS Executive, 2000: para 5.6.2.

55 NHS Executive, West Midlands. *Report of a review of the research framework in North Staffordshire Hospital NHS Trust* (Griffiths Inquiry). Birmingham: NHS Executive, 2000.

56 R v Cambridge HA Ex p. B (No.1) [1995] 1 WLR 898 at 903, [1995] 2 All ER 129, [1995] 1 FLR 1056, CA.

57 Ham C, Pickard S. *Tragic choices in health care. The case of child B*. London: King's Fund, 1998: xvi.

10: Health care in schools

10.1 School health services

Together with teaching and other school staff, school health services aim to:

- achieve the best possible level of health (mental and physical) and social wellbeing, currently and in the future for all children of school age; and
- work in partnership with children, parents and teachers to enable children to benefit fully from education.[1]

Their activities include child health surveillance, health interviews, health promotion, immunisation, child protection, liaison with parents, teachers and others involved in the child's care and drop-in sessions for children and parents.[2] The school doctor or nurse is involved in establishing whether there are any factors in a child's health that impede his or her ability to learn, and in advising whether children have illnesses that may pose a risk to other people.[3] Links with primary care through local GPs and practice nurses can ensure that children receive integrated care at school.

Services, particularly those for young children, have been criticised in the recent past, however, for being inaccessible, giving poor opportunities during consultations for children to raise issues and a lack of consent for routine examinations.[4] Although over the last few years there has been a trend towards more proactive services that better recognise the rights of children, improvement is hampered by a lack of resources and facilities.

Awareness by health services and local authorities of these potential problem areas can lead to improvement. Steps should be taken to ensure that the service's accommodation is appropriate for the provision of, for example, confidential health services. The function and activities of health professionals in schools should be clearly promoted to children and parents. Health professionals should look for signs that children want to raise issues during consultations, and should seek to involve both children and their parents. Lay and professional staff, local authorities and governing bodies should work together on local protocols for sharing information, and to ensure that contracts of employment reflect professional obligations. The BMA has worked with other bodies representing community health practitioners and published a document that presents an optimal view of the school health service and describes what is achieved in the best centres and what can be achieved with drive, commitment, enthusiasm and the support of primary care.[5] It identifies needs to: recognise the specialist nature of the school health service; improve the quality and take-up of training, and develop close working relationships with psychologists, paediatric nurses, dieticians, speech therapists, physiotherapists and social workers.

The BMA finds that the dilemmas of health professionals in schools are most common where lay staff ask them to act contrary to their professional obligations or to take on a role other than providing health care. In the past schools have sometimes sought to include in contracts of employment a requirement for school nurses to disclose information about all consultations to the school's head-teacher. Health care staff are also sometimes asked to become involved with screening children for evidence of drug misuse. The following sections address these and other potential areas of difficulty or misunderstanding and offer some guidance. Health professionals may also seek advice from professional, regulatory and indemnifying bodies.

10.2 Confidentiality

The duty of confidentiality that health professionals owe children, including those living away from the family home at residential schools, is as great as that owed to any other person.[6] That duty may only be breached where there is an overwhelming reason to do so, for example if the child or another person is at grave risk of serious harm if information is not disclosed. Where there is a need to disclose, the child concerned should be encouraged to agree to the disclosure following discussion about what information needs to be disclosed, to whom, why and what might happen as a result. Only if discussing disclosure with the child would itself cause serious harm might it be justifiable to disclose information without the child's knowledge or consent. Such situations are rare and are discussed in more detail in chapter 4.

Efforts should be made to promote the message about confidentiality to all children and young people. There is evidence to show that the major deterrent to young people asking for sexual health advice from their family doctor is anxiety about confidentiality, particularly where the doctor has close contact with other family members.[7] Such fears might be shared by children thinking about using a school health service if they believe disclosure to teaching staff or parents is routine. The confidential nature of the school health service, and also of other health care providers, should be promoted so that children and their parents understand what is available. A toolkit for general practice, giving advice about confidentiality and young people and suggesting strategies for informing young people of their rights, is published by Brook Advisory Centres, in association with the British Medical Association, the Royal College of General Practitioners and the Royal College of Nursing.[8] Schools are ideally placed to explain to children their rights to seek confidential access to health services and information, and may also find the information in the toolkit helpful.

In schools, it is usually the case that parents and relevant teaching staff are informed when an accident or injury occurs. Some such incidents will be immediately apparent to teachers in contact with the child, who may take responsibility for informing parents. It can be argued that health professionals in boarding schools cannot be expected to keep confidential, health information that would be apparent to parents if the child was living at home. For example, if a child suffers an injury that is visible to anybody who comes into contact with him or her, it could be argued that the fact of injury is not confidential. Keeping parents informed of such health matters may be necessary in order to protect parents' rights to family life (see chapters 2 and 3).[9]

Usually it is in the child's interests to inform parents and his or her consent should be sought to that end. Professional guidance states, however, that doctors must not disclose any personal information about their patients that they learn in their professional capacity and this would be particularly relevant if the information were sensitive or personal.[10] In most cases children will be willing to allow their doctor to contact their parents. Where they are not, children should be aware that teaching staff are likely to contact parents in the case of immediately apparent illness or injury.

As well as being kept informed by school staff about their child's health, parents with parental responsibility also have a statutory right of access to their child's health records, in certain circumstances. This includes the records of the school health service. Where the child is capable of giving consent to parental access, it can occur only with that agreement. If the child lacks the necessary capacity, access can be given if it is in the child's best interests. Information previously given in the expectation that it would be kept confidential should not be revealed, nor the results of investigations or examinations that the child thought were confidential at the time they were conducted. Access to records is covered in greater detail in chapter 4.

10.2.1 Inspection and monitoring of standards

Schools are inspected to monitor the standards achieved by children and the quality of learning and teaching. Problems may arise if inspectors wish to see records maintained by schools that contain health information. For example, teachers may keep records relating to the physical or mental health of students if it is relevant to the provision of education. Health professionals working in schools should ensure that lay staff are aware of the sensitive nature of health information and the need to keep it confidential as far as possible.

Teachers and carers should be encouraged to resist passing personal health information to inspectors. Whilst there may be grounds for confirming, for example, that schools are keeping records of health information necessary to support teachers' abilities to meet children's educational needs, it is generally inappropriate to pass details of such records to inspectors. If external investigations of standards of health care are needed, parents and children need to know and consent needs to be sought for access to records. Only in the most exceptional of circumstances, for example to prevent serious harm to others, should a refusal to allow access be overridden.

The GMC also requires doctors to monitor and maintain awareness of the quality of care being provided.[11] This should include taking part in regular and systematic clinical audit. Where doctors are working alone in schools, it may be helpful to involve colleagues from other schools or the doctor's own practice in audit that uses anonymous data. As in all areas of practice, patients should generally be aware that audit is carried out, and be told of their right to refuse to allow their information to be used for this purpose.

10.2.2 Disclosure of information to schools

General practice surgeries are sometimes contacted by schools checking up on pupils. It is an inappropriate breach of confidentiality for practices to reveal (without appropriate consent) whether or not a young person had an appointment on a particular day to establish whether he or she was playing truant, although the doctor may wish to discuss it with a pupil if medical appointments are given as a repeated excuse. Confidentiality may only be breached where there is an overwhelming public interest (see chapter 4).

10.3 Consent

Being resident away from the parental home, for example at boarding school, does not alter who can, in law, authorise or refuse treatment on behalf of a child. Competent young people, those with parental responsibility and a court may authorise a doctor to provide medical treatment and, as chapters 2 and 3 have shown, any person who has care of a child may also do "what is reasonable in all the circumstances of the case for the purpose of safeguarding or promoting the child's welfare".[12] This includes giving consent to necessary medical treatment, but is unlikely to cover non-urgent or prophylactic medical interventions. Parents may also arrange for certain aspects of parental responsibility to be met by somebody acting on the parents' behalf.[13]

Schools sometimes ask parents to confirm, in writing, that they are content for the school to take necessary action if it is not possible to contact the parents: this might be, for example, taking the child to a nearby hospital when away on a school trip. Although there is no legal requirement for the parents' permission, it is a way of ensuring that they are aware how the school deals with emergencies.

10.3.1 Consent to school medical examinations

School medical examinations are an essential part of the health service's role in preventive medicine. Examinations are carried out when children first enter school at age five, and again at age 13 or 14, with opportunities for other general or specific interventions between these times.

The form of consent required in order to carry out a routine medical examination of primary school children may raise dilemmas. Throughout this book the importance of involving parents in health care has been stressed, and it would be unfortunate if it became in any way routine for children to be seen in school without consent from parents. For medical assessments, the presence of parents provides a good safeguard, although this must be viewed together with the right of young people to confidentiality and to give consent for themselves.[14]

10.3.2 Implied consent for immunisation

Consent can be taken to be implied when patients (or those giving consent on behalf of children) understand what is being proposed, understand that they have a right to refuse and make no objection. In recent years, immunisation campaigns in some areas have been undertaken on this basis, with parents being given the opportunity to "opt out" rather than being required to give explicit consent. Doctors may only rely on implied consent if they are sure that the person concerned has definitely seen and understood the relevant information. Where there is any doubt, additional efforts should be made to ensure that there is no objection. Parents must be informed when immunisation is being carried out, and invited to give their permission. It may be ethically and legally justifiable, however, to proceed without their knowledge or consent where a competent child gives valid consent.

As well as consent from parents, the nature and purpose of the immunisation should be explained to all children who are then invited to agree. If competent young people refuse, doctors should consider whether the benefits to the child of having the immunisation outweigh the harm of overriding a competent refusal; they should also consider whether they need to seek legal advice. This process involves discussion with parents and the child, to see whether a compromise solution can be reached.

Some children may refuse, for example, because they don't want their friends to see them cry. Having the immunisation outside school hours, or at their GP surgery might be acceptable alternatives for these children. As previous chapters have discussed, doctors are unwilling to impose treatment on competent children who refuse unless there is good reason (see in particular section 6.1). There is a strong moral imperative to respect a competent refusal where doing so does not have serious consequences for the health or wellbeing of the child.

General consent for immunisation is sometimes sought from parents when their child begins boarding school. The Medical Officers of Schools Association (MOSA) suggests a standard consent form that parents sign indicating agreement "that the school medical officer may carry out such immunisations against tetanus, poliomyelitis, measles, mumps and rubella (German measles) as he deems necessary".[15] While discussion of these matters can be useful to ascertain parents' general views on immunisations, children should still be asked for consent. Parents should also understand that their decision when children first go to school is not immutable and that they may contact the school health service if their views change.

10.4 Medicines

Many children require the routine use of medicines, such as reliever inhalers for asthma, insulin for diabetes or rectal diazepam for epilepsy. Where there is no health professional providing cover throughout the whole school day, this raises questions of who is responsible for administering the medicines, and the responsibilities of teaching staff or other lay staff if children administer them themselves. It is desirable for children with long term recurring health problems such as these to be accommodated within school so that their education is not disrupted. For this to be done, however, proper and clearly understood arrangements for administration of medicines must be made. Parents should be encouraged to provide maximum support and assistance in helping the school accommodate the pupil, and jointly with the head-teacher should reach agreement on the school's role in helping with the child's medical needs.

Teachers have a professional duty to protect the health and safety of pupils and a general legal duty of care, but their conditions of service do not include any legal or contractual obligation to administer medicine or to supervise a child taking medicine.[16] Teachers may be willing to do so, however, with support, guidance and training from a member of the school health service or another appropriate health professional.[17] It is helpful if local authorities formulate protocols for good communication to facilitate this.[18] Teachers and employers should have regard to their potential liabilities in such circumstances.

Children, their parents, teachers and health professionals should work together to establish the best way to meet the child's needs. This might involve self administration of medication or parental supervision. Ideally doctors should prescribe for children so the need for medicines to be given during school hours is avoided. For example, if medicines need to be administered on a twice-daily basis, this can be done at home. Where administration at school is unavoidable, it is good practice to encourage even young pupils to manage their own medication where they can be trusted to do so.[19] Practical solutions that ensure the best possible care for the child without imposing unnecessary burdens on staff are the aim.

Guidance for schools on the storage and administration of medicines in schools is available from the Department for Education and Employment and the Department of Health.[20] The head-teacher is responsible, and the guidance gives practical suggestions for keeping medication so that it is readily accessible but only to authorised individuals. The following general principles are relevant:

- school staff should generally not give non-prescribed medicines to children;
- pupils must have access to their medicine when required;
- schools should not store large volumes of medication and wherever possible, children should bring in the dose they require each day;
- stored medicines should note the name of the pupil, name and dose of the drug and frequency of administration;
- pupils should know where their own medication is stored and who holds the key;
- medication that pupils may require urgently, such as asthma inhalers should not be locked away;
- parents are responsible for the collection and disposal of unused medicines; and

- all school staff should be familiar with and follow precautions for hygiene and infection control.

The guidance also stresses the importance of discussing management of illness with parents, and seeking their permission for teachers to administer medication to children. Individual care plans should be drawn up for children who require support at school, taking account of the child's own ability to manage his or her health. The head-teacher, parents, child, class-teacher, care assistant, support and other school staff, the school health service, the GP and any other health professionals involved in the child's care may all need to contribute to a plan.

Where teaching staff are willing to administer, or to supervise the administration of, medicines:

- the employer should arrange appropriate training in conjunction with the health authority;
- staff should understand and respect the need for confidentiality;
- a child who refuses to take medication should not be forced, and the school should inform the child's parents;
- staff should be aware when it is appropriate to contact the emergency services;
- there should be support mechanisms in place so staff can call on a named professional for advice; and
- local policies should require the presence of two members of staff for the administration of intimate or invasive treatment, at least one of whom should be the same gender as the child.

10.5 Drug misuse

Statistics show a steady increase in the use of illegal drugs amongst school-age children.[21] As a measure to combat this, drug education is provided in schools throughout the UK, although this is controversial and there has been little rigorous evaluation of its impact to date.[22] Some schools, predominantly in the independent sector, have also introduced drugs testing policies.

Where schools do offer or require testing, it is essential that both pupils and their parents are aware of this. They should be clear in advance when testing might be provided, and that decisions about whether to undergo testing (and whether to share the results with their parents) will be made by competent young people. At the same time, information must be provided about why the school offers testing, with policies emphasising that it is part of the educative process and not something carried out for punitive purposes.

In response to this move by the independent sector, in 1995 MOSA issued guidelines for testing for substance misuse in schools.[23] A number of key points from this guidance are summarised below.

- Wherever possible, the school health service should not be involved in the testing process. This respects its caring and supportive role. The collecting officer should be an outsider paid a retainer by the school to undertake this specific task.
- MOSA considers random testing of young people to be unethical. Testing should be where there is cause to suspect the individual is misusing drugs.
- Written informed consent should be obtained for the collection and testing of samples. Even where young people have the competence to give consent themselves, it is desirable that parents are aware that testing is taking place.
- The results of tests are confidential and should not be disclosed beyond the school authority requiring the test.
- Clear policies should be in place regarding how to deal with results, including practical strategies for ensuring abstinence.

10.6 Summary

- Children should understand the role of the school health service, and know how they can get confidential help and advice.
- Parents should be well informed about the role of the school health service, and invited to participate in routine activities involving their children.
- Parents should understand the extent of the role of teaching staff in supporting children with health needs in school.
- School staff caring for children are entitled to give consent to essential medical treatment where this is reasonable and necessary to safeguard or promote a child's welfare.

References

1 British Paediatric Association. *Report of a joint working party on health needs of school age children.* London: BPA, 1995.

2 Royal College of Nursing. *Health needs of school age children. An RCN briefing paper.* London: RCN, 1996.

3 The National Union of Teachers issues guidance for situations where children have infectious diseases. National Union of Teachers. *Infectious diseases in schools.* London: NUT, in press.

4 Mayall B. *Children, health and the social order.* Buckingham: Open University Press, 1996.

5 British Association of Community Child Health, British Medical Association Committee for Public Health Medicine and Community Health, Community Practitioners and Health Visitors Association and Royal College of Nursing. *Promoting children's health — developing an effective school health service.* London: BMA, 1997.

6 Further advice on confidentiality is available in British Medical Association, Brook Advisory Centres, Family Planning Association, Health Education Authority, Royal College of General Practitioners. *Confidentiality and people under 16.* London: BMA, 1993; British Medical Association. *Confidentiality and disclosure of health information.* London: BMA, 1999.

7 Egg Research and Consultancy Ltd. *You think they won't tell anyone, well you HOPE they won't ... Do young people believe sex advice is confidential?* A report commissioned by Brook Advisory Centres and the Royal College of General Practitioners and funded by the Department of Health. London: Egg Research & Consultancy, 1999. Available from Brook Advisory Centres Head Office.

8 British Medical Association, Brook Advisory Centres, Royal College of General Practitioners, Royal College of Nursing. *Confidentiality and young people. Improving teenagers' uptake of health advice. A toolkit for general practices.* London: Brook Advisory Centres, 2000.

9 Human Rights Act 1998.

10 General Medical Council. *Confidentiality: protecting and providing information.* London: GMC, 2000.

11 General Medical Council. *Good medical practice.* London: GMC, 1998: para 7.

12 Children Act 1989 s3(5). The Children (Northern Ireland) Order 1995 art 6(5). Children (Scotland) Act 1991 s5(1).

13 Children Act 1989 s2(9). The Children (Northern Ireland) Order 1995 art 5(8). Children (Scotland) Act 1991 s3(5).

14 British Paediatric Association. *Report of a joint working party on heath needs of school age children.* London: BPA, 1995.

15 Medical Officers of Schools Association. *Handbook of school health*, 18th edition. Stoke-on-Trent: Trentham Books, 1998: 310.

16 Teachers should seek advice, for example the National Union of Teachers publishes a briefing paper on the legal position of teachers. National Union of Teachers. *Medicines in schools.* London: NUT, 1999.

17 Department of Education and Science. *Staffing for pupils with special educational needs (DES Circular 11/90).* London: DES, 1990.

18 British Medical Association Community Health Doctors' Subcommittee. *Medication in schools.* London: BMA, 1994.

19 Department for Education and Employment, Department of Health. *Supporting pupils with medical needs.* London: DfEE, 1996.

20 Ibid.

21 British Medical Association. *The misuse of drugs.* Amsterdam: Harwood Academic Publishers, 1997: 14—15.

22 British Medical Association. *The misuse of drugs.* Amsterdam: Harwood

Academic Publishers, 1997: 31.
23 Medical Officers of Schools Association. *Handbook of school health*, 18th edition. Stoke-on-Trent: Trentham Books, 1998: 133—5.

11: Summary of good practice

In the preceding chapters, ethical, legal and practical issues have been considered separately. In this section, advice about different aspects of the care and treatment of children is integrated to provide a brief overview, under several main headings. Nevertheless, this summary is not designed to be read in isolation from the rest of the book. Rather, it is intended to highlight some of the main points that are considered in more depth in individual chapters. Doctors are also reminded of their obligations under the Human Rights Act 1998, which requires doctors, in all decision making, to have regard to whether their actions involve a person's human rights and, if so, whether those rights can legitimately be interfered with. Where it is clear that decision making might be affected by the Act, this has been noted in the text of the preceding chapters. The chapters shown in square brackets after the paragraphs below direct the reader to the more detailed discussion.

11.1 Decision making, information sharing, the child and the family

11.1.1 Involving children and young people in decision making

The development of a trusting relationship and good communication between health professionals and their patients are fundamental aspects of good practice. A good relationship between a health team and a child patient should establish a lifelong pattern of mutual trust and candour. As soon as they are able to communicate and participate in the decisions that affect them, children should be encouraged to express their views, ask questions and discuss their health worries. Nevertheless, young patients themselves should be able to set the pace for discussion. Sensitivity is required to ensure that they are not overwhelmed with information but given the time they need to absorb it. Health professionals should act as patient advocates and ensure the participation of children and young people in all aspects of decision making. This should be seen as the norm. If children are excluded from decision making, there must be justification for that stance. Wherever possible, however, children and young people should not have to take decisions alone but should be able to take them with support. Decision making should be family-centred. [Chapter 1]

11.1.2 Provision of information and truth-telling

Some children may not want to have full information or, they may need time to adjust to one aspect of the situation before receiving more details. Each patient is an individual and is entitled to be given information in a manner that is accessible and appropriate according to his or her level of understanding. Parents may try to insist on secrecy in order to protect their children from painful facts. This situation poses difficult dilemmas that need to be carefully worked through with the family in the light of the circumstances of the case. On the whole, we are against the withholding of information if the child seems willing to know it, even where parents request secrecy. We strongly advise against telling children lies in response to a clear question. In our view, questions should always be answered as frankly and as sensitively as possible: where there is uncertainty about the diagnosis, treatment or likely outcome, this should be acknowledged. [Chapters 1 and 5]

11.1.3 Children's refusal of information

It is unusual for children to refuse information unless they think that doing so helps others, such as their parents, to maintain a sense of "normality" in the face of serious illness. Children and young people should be encouraged to make all those decisions that they feel comfortable with and able to make. Wherever possible, decision making should not be hurried and patients should be given full opportunity to reflect, obtain more information and discuss the options in a supportive environment. If children and young people appear unwilling to have information, the reason should be sought, in case it is based on an erroneous view or on the child's wish to help parents cope. The child's wishes should be respected but it should also be made clear, that there are always opportunities for the child to change his or her mind and to be more involved in decision making. [Chapter 5]

11.1.4 Consent to treatment

The following are legally entitled to give consent to the medical treatment of a person under 18:

- a competent child;
- a parent or other person or agency with parental responsibility;
- a court;
- an appointed proxy (in Scotland where the patient is over 16 and unable to make decisions for him or herself); or
- a person caring for a child but only if it is reasonable in the circumstances to safeguard or promote the child's welfare.

In order for the consent of a young person to be authoritative, he or she must understand the implications of, and have appropriate information about, what is involved in the proposed treatment, the possible alternatives and the likely effects of non-treatment. [Chapters 2 and 3]

11.1.5 Involving families

The advice in this book consistently reinforces the message that the views of children and young people about their own health and treatment are extremely important. This is not to deny or underemphasise the key role of parents and the wider family. In the vast majority of cases, parents are the best and most appropriate people to take decisions for young children. As the child develops, he or she should gradually acquire a greater role in the decision — even to the point where mature children can legally and ethically exclude their parents from decision making. Nevertheless, when the patient is a person under the age of 18, it is desirable that parents or other people with parental responsibility provide support throughout the decision making and treatment process, but this must be balanced with the child's right to confidentiality. The younger and less experienced the patient is, the greater the role of the family in decision making. [Chapters 1, 2 and 3]

11.1.6 Parental responsibility

The law and medical ethics give parents and people with parental responsibility a set of duties in relation to children. This entails that they be given full and relevant information (unless the rules of confidentiality owed to the patient prohibit this) to enable them to make the best decision for and with their child. The state also has legal and moral obligations for the welfare of minors, which means that society has a clear duty to intervene if children and young people are avoidably put at risk of harm. It frequently falls to health professionals to carry out this duty to act in cases where neglect or abuse are suspected or where the health team simply considers that parents, possibly from a well-intentioned motive, are making treatment decisions that may harm children. In such cases, the courts may need to be involved. [Chapters 2, 3 and 4]

11.1.7 Emergencies

Where consent is unavailable, for example in an emergency when the patient is unable to communicate his or her wishes and where nobody with parental responsibility is available, it is legally and ethically appropriate for health professionals to proceed with treatment necessary to preserve the life, health or wellbeing of the patient. An emergency is best described as a situation where the requirement for treatment is so pressing that there is not time to refer the matter to court.

If such an emergency involves administering a treatment to which the child and/or family is known to object, for example the administration of blood to a Jehovah's Witness, viable alternatives should be explored if time allows. In extreme situations, however, health professionals are advised to take all essential steps to stabilise the patient. Legal advice may be needed once emergency action has been taken. (Health professionals should note however, that the law is likely to take a different view if an advance refusal by an adult is not implemented where relevant to the circumstances.) [Chapters 2, 3 and 6]

11.2 Competence and maturity in children and young people

11.2.1 Age and "maturity"

Age is not the most important factor in whether children may make their own decisions. Competence and "maturity" are more relevant. The ability of children and young people to make valid decisions is frequently underestimated. Children who have already experienced illness and medical treatment often have maturity beyond that normally expected for their age. This means that health professionals must be alert to the fact that some children are as able as many adults to make difficult treatment decisions. Nor is it appropriate to rely on assessments of competence made earlier, as children are constantly changing and developing. [Chapter 5]

11.2.2 Competence

Competence is function-specific. This entails health professionals assessing a patient's level of understanding in relation to the particular task in hand. Whilst some children clearly lack competence because of immaturity, health professionals should not judge the ability of a particular child on the basis of his or her age. Health professionals should take all reasonable steps to enhance the ability of children to participate in decision making, and encourage them to do so. [Chapter 5]

11.3 Promoting benefit, avoiding harm: the "best interests" criterion

11.3.1 Best interests

The patient's best interests is the paramount criterion in decision making with children and young people. The term "best interests" is a slippery one that is sometimes interpreted to mean providing any treatment that might prolong life or prevent deterioration in health regardless of the patient's and the family's views. Once they understand the options, patients are usually the best arbiters of their own interests. The individual's overall welfare should be the paramount consideration and listening to minors' views is conducive to promoting their welfare in the widest sense. Any assessment of best interests should be pursued in a holistic manner, taking into account the various physical, emotional, social, cultural and psychological needs of the whole person. In some situations, non-treatment is entirely compatible with the patient's overall best interests. Providing treatment to a competent young person against his or her wishes may require the approval of a court, particularly if providing it requires the use of restraint or containment. The harm caused by violating a competent child's choice must be balanced against the harm caused by failing to treat. [Chapters 1 and 6]

11.3.2 Benefit and harm

The arguments that need to be considered in relation to an assessment of benefit and harm are very similar to those involved in an assessment of best interests. It is important that the concepts of harm and benefit are seen in a wider context than that of purely medical factors. Patients are arguably not benefited when invasive treatments are carried out contrary to their will and at variance with their own firmly held wishes. A difficulty for health professionals, however, is that of ascertaining whether the patient's decision is a well considered and valid one or an understandable but possibly hasty reaction to an unfamiliar situation. In previous chapters we have included examples of cases where the courts judged that a young person lacked sufficient competence and judgment to refuse life-prolonging treatment when an urgent decision had to be made. [Chapters 1, 2 and 3]

11.4 Circumstances where dilemmas arise

11.4.1 Disputes

Dilemmas usually arise because there is some form of dispute about the best course of action to be followed. Competent children may disagree with their parents or with the courts, as examples in previous chapters indicate. Or the family members may all be in agreement but oppose the treatment plan suggested by the health team. Health professionals must focus on the overall best interests of the patient even when this creates tension with other family members. Many disputes arise because of poor communication and all efforts should be made to avoid this. An independent second opinion may also be helpful in resolving some disagreements but ultimately, some may have to be resolved by the courts. [Chapter 6]

11.4.2 A child's refusal of treatment

Young and immature children may refuse treatment without fully understanding the implications and this is not a valid decision. Morally, it is a different matter if the patient understands what is at stake. When medical treatment has been recommended and is met by a refusal from a competent child or young person, this is always a serious situation that needs to be given very careful attention. The reasons should be discussed to ensure that the refusal is not based on inaccurate perceptions. In some circumstances, non-treatment — even where the treatment is potentially life-prolonging — is consistent with the patient's overall best interests. In these cases, there are good moral arguments for following the patient's wishes, particularly if this is also the view of the family (but see also section 11.4.3. [Chapters 1 and 6]

11.4.3 The parents' role

In England, Wales and Northern Ireland a refusal of treatment by someone under 18 can be overruled by a court or by a person with parental responsibility. Health professionals faced with an informed refusal of a treatment they believe to be beneficial may need to take legal advice, although it is clear that people with parental responsibility can give legally valid consent on behalf of a child or young person. Therefore, the law and the ethical stance deemed most appropriate throughout this book may seem at odds on this issue of refusal since the refusal is seen as significant but legally it can be overruled. In practice, however, this distinction is not always a sharp one. Even though importance should be given to a child's informed refusal, health professionals and society generally are extremely reluctant to allow a life to be lost or health risks to be taken by a young person if this is avoidable. Because harm to a child is universally seen as a tragic occurrence, every effort is usually made to ensure that medical treatment that could be beneficial is not left untried. [Chapters 2 and 6]

In Scotland, if a competent child refuses consent to treatment, from current case law and statute it seems likely that this refusal of consent cannot be overridden by any other person, carer or court. This matter is not beyond doubt and legal advice should be sought where such situations arise. [Chapter 3]

11.4.4 Parental insistence on active treatment

Legally and ethically, treatment should only be offered when it is perceived to be in the best interests of the patient. When children are very seriously ill, however, families often find it difficult to accept that further treatment may be futile and there may be a perception that families derive comfort from the continuation of some form of active treatment rather than the transition to palliative care. Clearly, however, although support to the family and continuing dialogue are very important, the patient's interests must be the paramount consideration. [Chapter 6]

11.4.5 The courts as final arbiter

Furthermore, even though the refusal of even a competent person under 18 can, in certain circumstances, legally be overridden by somebody with parental responsibility or a court, in cases where the patient, the family and the health team clearly indicate that they have considered all the arguments and reached a consensus to support the patient's or parents' refusal, this is likely to influence the court's decision. [Chapters 2, 3 and 6]

11.4.6 Distinction between authority to treat and obligation to treat

Just because parental or court consent has been given and can legally override a child's refusal of treatment, this does not mean that it is necessarily in the child's best interests for the treatment to proceed. Health professionals have obligations over and above the requirement to obtain valid consent and must weigh the benefits of providing the treatment against the harm caused by overriding a competent child's refusal. Nevertheless, the moral imperative to provide treatment against a young person's wishes is greater where there are good grounds to assume that the treatment would actually achieve a significant prolongation or enhancement of the patient's life. In other words, a young patient's refusal is more likely to determine the outcome in situations where there is doubt that the treatment could make a really significant difference. [Chapters 2, 3 and 6]

11.5 Withdrawing and withholding treatment

There is no legal or ethical obligation for health professionals to provide medical treatment that cannot achieve its clinical aim, or that does not provide an overall benefit to the child. In deciding whether treatment should be begun or stopped, health professionals should assess the relevant clinical factors and other vital factors, such as the wishes of the patient and family. Support for the child and family is essential throughout the process of deciding about the provision of life-prolonging treatment, and during and following its implementation. Constant review of the child's condition is essential, and all decisions and changes to the child's circumstances should be documented in the health record. [Chapter 6]

11.5.1 Disagreements about when to cease treatment

All efforts should be made to overcome disagreements about treatment. Assessment of the benefits a treatment offers and balancing potential benefits in the light of the wishes of children and their families is a part of routine practice. The decisions become particularly difficult where the benefits and burdens are finely balanced, for example where there is only a very slim chance that a very invasive treatment will give some chance of improvement in a serious condition, or when agreement about how to proceed cannot be reached by the family and health care team. [Chapter 6]

11.6 Confidentiality and control of information

11.6.1 Children's confidentiality

Children and young people are entitled to medical confidentiality on the same grounds as other patients. This means that their rights are not absolute but can only generally be overridden when there is a clear justification, such as the risk of significant harm. Where there is an exceptional reason justifying disclosure without consent, children should be told that their secrets cannot be kept. In the absence of any such reason justifying disclosure, they should be encouraged but not forced to share their health information with parents. [Chapter 4]

11.6.2 Confidentiality of other family members

Because children's rights and their protection are seen as having such vital importance, the rights of other family members are sometimes forgotten. In particular, this can occur in relation to child protection inquiries. Health professionals are sometimes asked to disclose the health records of all family members without the knowledge or consent of the individuals concerned. Although no person is entitled to absolute and inflexible confidentiality, no person's rights can be simply ignored for the sake of convenience or to avoid the embarrassment of telling the family that child protection concerns have been raised. In exceptional cases, the confidentiality of any person can be overridden for the greater public good and this is usually interpreted as being the case where a child's safety may be at risk. Nevertheless, where it is feasible to ask people's permission for disclosure, this should be the norm. [Chapter 4 and Appendix 1]

11.6.3 Access to health records

Competent children and young people control access to their own health records. They have rights to see their records themselves and can allow or prohibit access by other people, including parents. People with parental responsibility also have a statutory right of access to their children's health records where the child is unable to give consent and disclosure is in the child's interests. [Chapter 4]

11.6.4 Access to information by schools

Schools and people looking after children should not generally have more rights over information about children than parents themselves have. As mentioned above, competent children and young people can refuse their parents access to their health records in certain circumstances. Schools should respect the confidentiality of children. In exceptional cases, there may be grounds for requesting disclosure of health information in order to protect the child or other people from harm, such as where an infectious disease may be present or the child's activities put other people at risk of serious harm. Where schools are likely to require disclosure in some circumstances or have a policy of drugs testing pupils, it is important that children and their families are aware in advance of these policies. [Chapter 10]

11.7 Mental disorder

The fundamental principles of good practice are the same in mental health care as in other forms of treatment. In particular,

SUMMARY OF GOOD PRACTICE

health professionals should ensure that:

- care is provided consensually wherever possible and patient autonomy respected;
- minors' views are always taken into account;
- information is provided and there is effective communication;
- all patients are as involved as possible in developing their own care plan;
- care and treatment are non-discriminatory and respect diversity;
- care is provided in the least restrictive setting possible;
- treatment involves the least possible segregation from family, friends and school;
- where possible, families are involved in decisions about therapy; and
- patient confidentiality is respected.

Informal care should be considered before recourse to compulsory care and treatment should be evidence-based. [Chapter 7]

11.8 Research and sensitive or innovative procedures

Views about what constitute sensitive or controversial procedures change over time. Parental consent is not always sufficient to justify an intervention that does not demonstrably appear to be in the child's own interests. If in doubt, doctors should seek legal advice. [Chapters 8 and 9]

11.8.1 Informed consent

As in other cases, consent should be sought from competent children and young people. Legally, parents and people with parental responsibility can give proxy consent to procedures that are in the child's interests but cannot validly authorise procedures that are not. Where doctors modify a standard procedure or introduce a new treatment, they should inform patients and their parents of the reasons and whether there are foreseeable variations in the risks involved. If serious disputes arise in connection with controversial treatments, the courts may have to decide where the child's interests lie. Some procedures are sufficiently controversial for the courts to require consent from both parents. [Chapters 8 and 9]

11.8.2 Treatment to benefit other people

Medical interventions may be ethically acceptable when they are neutral. That is to say, even if they are not directly in the child's own interests, they may be permissible if not clearly contrary to those best interests. Informed parental consent, and wherever possible the child's own agreement, are required in such cases. [Chapter 8]

11.8.3 Audit of new procedures

Health professionals must monitor closely whether the outcomes from their treatment patterns fall below the success rate gained by other practitioners. If so, attention needs to be given urgently to investigating the reasons for this.

Once success rates of a new procedure appear hopeful, a formal research protocol should be drawn up for appraisal by a research ethics committee. Doctors should not continue indefinitely with an innovative procedure that has not been tested against standard options. [Chapter 9]

11.8.4 Research

Any intervention or research whose goal is not that of directly benefiting the child must carry no more than minimal risk; it must not entail pain for the child; informed parental and research ethics committee agreement must be obtained, and the child should not be included contrary to his or her wishes. [Chapter 9]

11.9 Further advice

Where there is any doubt, doctors should seek advice from their professional, regulatory and indemnifying bodies. The contact details of some relevant organisations are given in appendix 2.

Appendix 1

Examination or assessment for child protection purposes

Chapter 4 discusses the disclosure and use of information where this is necessary to protect a child from serious harm. This appendix describes the doctor's role in obtaining consent for an examination or assessment; the permission that is required if proceedings under the Children Act 1989 (or its equivalents in other UK jurisdictions) have been initiated; what to do if the child refuses examination or assessment, and the role of the expert witness.

The need for consent

Except in an emergency, any examination or assessment that involves physical contact with the child requires consent (from a competent child, a parent or another person with parental responsibility), or authorisation from a court. Even if assessment does not involve physical contact (for example an interview as part of a psychological or psychiatric assessment), consent is needed.[1]

As in other contexts, any person with parental responsibility may provide consent. The opposition of one person with parental responsibility does not prevent a valid consent being given by another. Therefore, for example, if there are concerns about the possibility of abuse by a young child's father, it may be possible to obtain consent for an assessment from the child's mother. If an assessment is necessary, and no valid consent can be obtained, legal advice must be sought and it may be necessary to apply to the courts for authorisation of an assessment.

Requirements for valid consent to a child protection assessment

To obtain legally valid consent, it is necessary for the person giving consent to be informed of the nature and purpose of the proposed assessment. The person giving consent should not be deceived or misled about the purpose of an assessment. Being open about the purpose is clearly necessary when an assessment is requested by a statutory agency responsible for child protection (for example, social services or the police).

At the earliest stages of a case, and before other professional agencies are involved, abuse or neglect may be just one of several possible explanations for a child's condition. Where an assessment is to evaluate the child's health needs, it may be counterproductive to mention prematurely that abuse is the possible cause. Therefore, the amount of information that must be disclosed when seeking consent is a matter for careful professional judgment, taking account of the level of professional concern at the time. Guidance on this has been issued by the Department of Health, the British Medical Association and the Conference of Medical Royal Colleges, which provides a description of the development of professional concern:

Child abuse may present in a variety of complex and intricate ways; for example as a suspicion when signs and symptoms are present but their significance is unclear, with clear physical signs or with an allegation or a disclosure. Where there is clear evidence of abuse or if an allegation has been made there should be no delay in referring this to the statutory agencies.

Where uncertainty exists doctors will often find it helpful to test out professional hypotheses before initial concerns about child abuse are shared with non-medical colleagues. Doctors should clarify their own thoughts about a particular case, and with advice as appropriate from senior or more experienced colleagues, reach a critical threshold of professional concern. When a critical threshold of professional concern is reached doctors must be prepared to share these concerns with the statutory agencies for further evaluation and discussion **within a time frame which is not detrimental to the child's interests.**

The critical threshold of professional concern is a matter of individual professional judgement made by someone with experience in child protection matters and will inevitably vary

between professionals and between situations. Training,
supervision and experience will be crucial, however, in
determining where this threshold is set.[2]

Once a critical threshold of professional concern has been reached, it becomes necessary to share information and concerns with other agencies before further assessments take place. Detailed guidance on the role of different agencies, including medical professionals, within the child protection systems is contained in various Department of Health publications.[3]

The need to avoid unnecessary assessments

The courts have emphasised that it is harmful for children to be exposed to an unnecessarily large number of assessments. For example, in the case of *Re CS*, the High Court heard that a child had been subjected to 12 intimate physical examinations by the same doctor.[4] Mrs Justice Bracewell said:

By reason of the failure of the court to control the examination
of [the child], she was, in my judgment, subjected to abusive
intimate examinations on more occasions than could possibly
be justified.[5]

Once legal proceedings have begun, the court is responsible for deciding whether an assessment is required for the purposes of the proceedings, having regard to the child's welfare. Nevertheless, there is a danger that children may be repeatedly assessed *before* court proceedings have been initiated. For example, one parent may be convinced that the other parent is abusive, and be determined to seek evidence to confirm this. In other cases, a parent may agree to a series of assessments at the request of a local authority, because of a fear that the local authority will initiate care proceedings if consent is not granted. In such situations, professionals must exercise independent judgment in deciding whether a further assessment is necessary and in the child's interests.

Where there are concerns that inappropriate and unnecessary assessments are being carried out, it has been suggested that an order could be sought from the court, prohibiting a parent from granting consent for further assessments.[6]

The role of the court under the Children Act

Once legal proceedings under the Children Act (or its equivalent in other UK jurisdictions[7]) have been initiated, the court is responsible for making decisions about the conduct of the proceedings, including whether any assessments should be carried out. The Family Proceedings Rules 1991 state:

> *No person may, without the leave of the court, cause the child to be medically or psychiatrically examined, or otherwise assessed, for the purpose of the preparation of expert evidence for use in the proceedings.*[8]

Therefore, before undertaking an assessment for the purpose of legal proceedings, medical professionals should confirm that the court has granted permission (known as "leave") for the assessment. Obviously this requirement does not prevent any assessment that is necessary for the child's health, since this is not undertaken for the purpose of the preparation of expert evidence. In addition, when the court makes certain orders, it can positively direct that an assessment should take place, or direct that there is to be no examination of the child. For example the Children Act states:

> *(6)   Where the court makes an interim care order, or interim supervision order, it may give such directions (if any) as it considers appropriate with regard to the medical or psychiatric examination or other assessment of the child; but if the child is of sufficient understanding to make an informed decision he may refuse to submit to the examination or other assessment.*
>
> *(7)   A direction under subsection (6) may be to the effect that there is to be–*
> *(a) no such examination or assessment; or*
> *(b) no such examination or assessment unless the court directs otherwise.*[9]

Similar provisions apply to emergency protection orders and child assessment orders.[10]

Refusal of examination

It is significant that the sections of the Children Act that allow the court to direct that an assessment should take place also state that a child who is of "sufficient understanding to make an informed decision" may refuse to submit to the examination or assessment (see chapters 2 and 3).[11] Therefore, even where an assessment has been specifically authorised by a court, it is still necessary to assess the level of the child's understanding, and to seek the child's agreement, before proceeding with the assessment (see chapter 5).

Recommendations concerning a child's refusal

Where a child refuses to cooperate with an assessment, there are several possibilities.

- It may be decided that assessment is impossible without the child's cooperation, or that it would be inappropriate to proceed in the face of the child's objections. In these circumstances, legal advice should be sought.
- It may be decided that the child lacks sufficient understanding to make an informed decision. An authorised assessment can lawfully proceed despite the child's objections, although health professionals may well be unwilling to proceed in such circumstances. If it is likely to be necessary to use force or sedatives to overcome the child's resistance, legal advice should be sought.
- It may be decided that the child is considered to have sufficient understanding to make an informed decision. In these circumstances, the court has no power under the Children Act to override the child's refusal. However, in the case of *South Glamorgan County Council* v *B*,[12] it was decided that the High Court exercising its "inherent jurisdiction" may authorise an assessment against the wishes of a competent child if the child would otherwise be likely to suffer "significant harm" (see section 2.2.2). This power is not available in magistrates' courts or county courts, and this precedent is unlikely to be followed in Scotland (see chapter 3).

Carrying out assessments of children against their wishes is very controversial. Such assessments are unlikely to be appropriate unless:

- there is a high probability that useful evidence can be obtained;
- the evidence cannot be obtained in any other way; and
- the benefit to the child from obtaining the evidence outweighs the burdens involved in imposing the assessment on the child.

The role of the expert witness

Specific guidance on providing expert evidence for courts is provided in the professional literature.[13] There are now also a large number of judicial decisions, where the courts have given guidance on the appointment of experts. The important points can be summarised, as below.[14]

Information to be provided to experts

- Experts should seek further information and documentation when required.
- Doctors who have prior clinical experience of a child should have all clinical materials in advance of the hearing for inspection by the court and other experts. This might include medical notes, hospital records, x-rays, photographs and correspondence.
- Experts who are to give evidence must be kept up to date with developments in the case relevant to their opinions and it is the duty of the solicitor instructing the expert to provide such information.

Duties of experts

- Expert evidence presented to the court should be, and should be seen to be, the independent product of the expert, uninfluenced by others. Experts should provide independent assistance to the court by objective unbiased opinion, in relation to matters within their expertise.
- Experts should state the facts or assumptions on which their opinions are based, and should not omit to consider material facts that detract from their conclusions.
- Experts should make it clear when a particular aspect is outside their expertise.
- If an expert opinion is not properly researched by reason of insufficient data, then this must be stated with an indication that the opinion is provisional.
- If at any time an expert changes his or her opinion on a material matter, this information must be communicated to the other parties, and, when appropriate, to the court.
- If an opinion is based, wholly or in part, on research conducted by others, this must be clearly set out in the report, the research relied on must be identified, and the expert must be prepared to justify the opinions expressed.

APPENDIX 1

Further advice

Further advice on these issues may be sought from professional, regulatory or indemnifying bodies.

References

1 The courts have stated that a decision whether a child should be interviewed is an aspect of parental responsibility and that therefore consent is needed. Re F (Minors) (Specific Issue: Child Interview), sub nom Re F (Minors) (Solicitors Interviews) [1995] 1 FLR 819, [1995] 2 FCR 200, CA. Re M (Minors: Interview), sub nom Re M (Minors) (Solicitors Interviews); Re M (Care: Leave to Interview Child) [1995] 1 FLR 825, [1995] 2 FCR 643, [1995] Fam Law 404.

2 Department of Health, British Medical Association, Conference of Medical Royal Colleges. *Child protection: medical responsibilities*. London: Department of Health, 1992: paras 2.4—2.6.

3 See for example, Department of Health, Home Office, Department for Education and Employment. *Working together to safeguard children*. London: The Stationery Office, 1999. Department of Health, British Medical Association, Conference of Medical Royal Colleges. *Child protection: medical responsibilities*. London: Department of Health, 1992.

4 Re CS (Expert Witnesses) [1996] 2 FLR 115.

5 Re CS (Expert Witnesses) [1996] 2 FLR 115 at 119.

6 D v D (County Court Jurisdiction: Injunctions) [1993] 2 FLR 802, [1994] Fam Law 8.

7 The Children (Northern Ireland) Order 1995. Children (Scotland) Act 1995.

8 Family Proceedings Rules (SI 1991/1247).

9 Children Act 1989 s38. The Children (Northern Ireland) Order 1995 art 57. The Children (Scotland) Act gives competent young people the right to refuse to submit to medical or psychiatric examination or other assessment that has been directed by the court or a children's hearing for the purpose of supervision requirement, assessment, protection or place of safety order. Children (Scotland) Act s90.

10 Children Act 1989 s43 and 44. The Children (Northern Ireland) Order 1995 art 62 and 63.

11 Children Act 1989 s38(6). The Children (Northern Ireland) Order 1995 art 57(6). Children (Scotland) Act 1995 s90.

12 South Glamorgan CC v B, sub nom South Glamorgan CC v W and B [1993] FLR 574, [1993] 1 FCR 626, [1993] Fam Law 398.

13 Royal College of Physicians. *Physical signs of sexual abuse in children*. London: RCP, 1997. See also Black D, Harris-Hendricks J, Wolkind S. *Child psychiatry and the law*, 3rd edition. London: Gaskell, 1998: chapters 3 and 4.

14 Children Act Advisory Committee. *1994/5 Report of the Children Act Advisory Committee*. London: Lord Chancellor's Department, 1996: 25—26.

Appendix 2

Useful addresses

British Association of Community Child Health
c/o Royal College of Paediatrics and Child Health,
50 Hallam Street, London W1W 6DE
Tel: 020 7307 5640, Fax: 020 7307 5601

British Association of Paediatric Surgeons
c/o Royal College of Surgeons of England,
35—43 Lincoln's Inn Fields, London WC2A 3PH
Tel: 020 7869 6915, Fax: 020 7869 6919
Email: adminsec@baps.org.uk
Internet: www.baps.org.uk

British Medical Association
BMA House, Tavistock Square, London WC1H 9JP
Tel: 020 7387 4499, Fax: 020 7383 6400
Email: enquiries@bma.org.uk
Internet: www.bma.org.uk

Brook Advisory Centres
421 Highgate Studios,
53—79 Highgate Road, London NW5 1TL
Tel: 020 7284 6040, Fax: 020 7284 6050
Email: information@brookcentres.org.uk
Internet: www.brook.org.uk

Children's Legal Centre
c/o University of Essex
Wivenhoe Park, Colchester, Essex CO4 3SQ
Tel: 01206 872466, Fax: 01206 874026
Email: clc@essex.ac.uk
Internet: www2.essex.ac.uk/clc

Children's Rights Alliance for England
(Incorporating the Children's Rights Development Unit and
Children's Rights Office)
319 City Road, London EC1V 1LJ
Tel: 020 7278 8222, Fax: 020 7278 9552
Email: info@crights.org.uk

Community Practitioners and Health Visitors Association
40 Bermondsey Street, London SE1 3UD
Tel: 020 7939 7000, Fax: 020 7403 2976
Internet: www.msfcphva.org

Council for Professions Supplementary to Medicine
Park House, 184 Kennington Park Road, London SE11 4BU
Tel: 020 7582 0866, Fax: 020 7820 9684
Internet: www.cpsm.org.uk

Department for Education and Employment
Sanctuary Buildings, Great Smith Street, London SW1P 3BT
Tel: 0870 001 2345, Fax: 020 7925 6971
Internet: www.dfee.gov.uk

Department of Education (Northern Ireland)
Rathgael House, Balloo Road, Bangor,
County Down BT19 7PR
Tel: 02891 279279, Fax: 02891 279100
Email: deni@nics.gov.uk
Internet: www.deni.gov.uk

Department of Health
Wellington House,
133—155 Waterloo Road, London SE1 8UG
Tel: 020 7972 2000
Internet: www.open.gov.uk/doh/dhhome.htm

Faculty of Pharmaceutical Medicine
1 St Andrew's Place, London NW1 4LB
Tel: 020 7224 0343, Fax: 020 7224 5381
Email: fpm@f-pharm-med.org.uk
Internet: www.f-pharm-med.org.uk

General Medical Council
178 Great Portland Street, London W1W 5JE
Tel: 020 7580 7642, Fax: 020 7915 3641
Email: gmc@gmc-uk.org
Internet: www.gmc-uk.org

Human Fertilisation and Embryology Authority
Paxton House, 30 Artillery Lane, London E1 7LS
Tel: 020 7377 5077, Fax: 020 7377 1871
Internet: www.hfea.gov.uk

Human Rights Task Force
Human Rights Unit, Home Office, Room 1075,
50 Queen Anne's Gate, London SW1H 9AT
Tel: 020 7273 2166, Fax: 020 7273 2045
Email: humanrightsunit@homeoffice.gsi.gov.uk
Internet: www.homeoffice.gov.uk/hract

Institute for Public Policy Research
30—32 Southampton Street, London WC2E 7RA
Tel: 020 7470 6100, Fax: 020 7470 6111
Email: postmaster@ippr.org.uk
Internet: www.ippr.org.uk

Institute of Child Health
30 Guilford Street, London WC1N 1EH
Tel: 020 7242 9789, Fax: 020 7831 0488
Internet: www.ich.ucl.ac.uk

Institute of Medical Illustrators
Bank Chambers, 48 Onslow Gardens,
London SW7 3AH
Internet: www.imi.org.uk

Jehovah's Witness Hospital Information Services
Watch Tower House, The Ridgeway, London NW7 1RN
Tel: 020 8906 2211, Fax: 020 8349 4545
Email: his@wtbts.org.uk
Internet: www.watchtower.org

Justice
59 Carter Lane, London EC4V 5AQ
Tel: 020 7329 5100, Fax: 020 7329 5055
Email: admin@justice.org.uk
Internet: www.justice.org.uk

Keeper's Office
Court of Session, Parliament House, Parliament Square,
Edinburgh EH1 1RQ
Tel: 0131 225 2595

Law Commission
Conquest House, 37—38 John Street, London WC1N 2BQ
Tel: 020 7453 1220, Fax: 020 7453 1297
Email: secretary.lawcomm@gtnet.gov.uk
Internet: www.lawcom.gov.uk

Law Society
13 Chancery Lane, London WC2A 1PL
Tel: 020 7242 1222, Fax: 020 7831 0344
Internet: www.lawsociety.org.uk

Law Society of Scotland
26 Drumsheugh Gardens, Edinburgh EH3 7YR
Tel: 0131 226 7411, Fax: 0131 225 2934
Email: lawscot@lawscot.org.uk
Internet: www.lawscot.org.uk

Medical Defence Union
230 Blackfriars Road, London SE1 8PG
Tel: 020 7202 1500, Fax: 020 7202 1666
Email: mdu@the-mdu.com
Internet: www.the-mdu.com

Medical and Dental Defence Union of Scotland
Mackintosh House, 120 Blythswood Street, Glasgow G2 4EA
Tel: 0141 221 5858, Fax: 0141 228 1208
Email: info@mddus.com
Internet: www.mddus.com

Medical Officers of Schools Association
c/o Dr Neil Arnott (Honorary Secretary),
The Amherst Medical Practice,
21 St Botolph's Road, Sevenoaks, Kent TN13 3AQ
Tel: 01732 459255, Fax: 01732 450751
Internet: www.mosa.org.uk

Medical Protection Society
33 Cavendish Square, London W1G 0PS
Tel: 0845 605 4000, Fax: 020 7399 1301
Email: info@mps.org.uk
Internet: www.mps.org.uk

Medical Research Council
20 Park Crescent, London W1B 1AL
Tel: 020 7636 5422, Fax: 020 7436 6179
Internet: www.mrc.ac.uk

Mental Health Act Commission
Maid Marian House,
56 Hounds Gate, Nottingham NG1 6BG
Tel: 0115 943 7100, Fax: 0115 943 7101
Email: chief.executive@mhac.trent.nhs.uk
Internet: www.mhac.trent.nhs.uk

Mental Welfare Commission for Scotland
K Floor, Argyle House,
3 Lady Lawson Street, Edinburgh EH3 9SH
Tel: 0131 222 6111, Fax: 0131 222 6112
Internet: www.mwcscot.org.uk

National Children's Bureau
8 Wakley Street, London EC1V 7QE
Tel: 020 7843 6000, Fax: 020 7278 9512
Internet: www.ncb.org.uk

Official Solicitor of the Supreme Court
81 Chancery Lane, London WC2A 1DD
Tel: 020 7911 7127, Fax: 020 7911 7105
Email: offsol@offsol.fsnet.co.uk
Internet: www.offsol.demon.co.uk
From April 2001, the Children and Family Court Advisory
and Support Service (CAFCASS) will take over the functions
of the Official Solicitor in respect of children.

Official Solicitor of the Supreme Court for Northern Ireland
Royal Courts of Justice, PO Box 410, Belfast BT1 3JF
Tel: 02890 235111, Fax: 02890 313793

Royal College of General Practitioners
14 Princes Gate, Hyde Park, London SW7 1PU
Tel: 020 7581 3232, Fax: 020 7225 3047
Email: info@rcgp.org.uk
Internet: www.rcgp.org.uk

Royal College of Nursing
20 Cavendish Square, London W1M 0AB
Tel: 020 7409 3333, Fax: 020 7647 3435
Internet: www.rcn.org.uk

Royal College of Obstetricians and Gynaecologists
27 Sussex Place, Regents Park, London NW1 4RG
Tel: 020 7772 6200, Fax: 020 7723 0575
Internet: www.rcog.org.uk

Royal College of Paediatrics and Child Health
50 Hallam Street, London W1N 6DE
Tel: 020 7307 5600, Fax: 020 7307 5601
Internet: www.rcpch.ac.uk

Royal College of Physicians
11 St Andrew's Place, London NW1 4LE
Tel: 020 7935 1174, Fax: 020 7487 5218
Email: info@rcplondon.ac.uk
Internet: www.rcplondon.ac.uk

Royal College of Physicians and Surgeons of Glasgow
232—242 St Vincent Street, Glasgow G2 5RJ
Tel: 0141 221 6072, Fax: 0141 221 1804
Internet: www.rcpsglasg.ac.uk

Royal College of Physicians of Edinburgh
9 Queen Street, Edinburgh EH2 1JQ
Tel: 0131 225 7324, Fax: 0131 220 3939
Internet: www.rcpe.ac.uk

Royal College of Psychiatrists
17 Belgrave Square, London SW1X 8PG
Tel: 020 7235 2351, Fax: 020 7245 1231
Email: rcpsych@rcpsych.ac.uk
Internet: www.rcpsych.ac.uk

Royal Courts of Justice
Strand, London WC1A 2LL
Tel: 020 7947 6000

Scottish Executive Education Department
Victoria Quay, Edinburgh EH6 6QQ
Tel: 0131 556 8400
Internet: www.scotland.gov.uk

Scottish Executive Health Department
St Andrew's House, Regent Road, Edinburgh EH1 3DG
Tel: 0131 556 8400
Internet: www.scotland.gov.uk

Scottish Executive Solicitors Office
Victoria Quay, Edinburgh EH6 6QQ
Tel: 0131 556 8400
Internet: www.scotland.gov.uk

Scottish Law Commission
140 Causewayside, Edinburgh EH9 1PR
Tel: 0131 668 2131, Fax: 0131 662 4900
Email: info@scotlawcom.gov.uk
Internet: www.scotlawcom.gov.uk

United Kingdom Central Council for Nursing,
Midwifery and Health Visiting
23 Portland Place, London W1N 4JT
Tel: 020 7637 7181, Fax: 020 7436 2924
Internet: www.ukcc.org.uk

World Medical Association
PO Box 63, 01212 Ferney-Voltaire Cedex, France
Tel: +33 (0)4 50 40 75 75, Fax: +33 (0)4 50 40 59 37
Email: info@wma.net
Internet: www.wma.net

Young Minds
102—108 Clerkenwell Road, London EC1M 5SA
Tel: 020 7336 8445, Fax: 020 7336 8446
Email: enquiries@youngminds.org.uk
Internet: www.youngminds.org.uk

Index

Note: The abbreviation EWNI is used to stand for the law regarding England, Wales and Northern Ireland.
Page numbers in **bold type** refer to entries in the final chapter, 'Summary of good practice'. Page numbers in *italics* refer to the Appendices.